Tooth & Gum Care

Densie Hatfield

American Family Health Institute™

SPRINGHOUSE CORPORATION
SPRINGHOUSE, PA.

Program Director
Stanley Loeb

Clinical Director
Barbara McVan, RN

Art Director
John Hubbard

Editors
Jay Hyams
Susan Cass
Kevin Law

Designer
Maria Errico

Editorial Services Manager
David Moreau

Senior Production Manager
Deborah Meiris

Production Coordinator
Sally Johnson

The charter of the American Family Health Institute is to research and produce high-quality publications that enhance the health of individuals and their families. Essential to health are physical, emotional, and social well-being, not just the absence of illness or infirmity. The Institute's Medical Board has produced the *Health and Fitness* books to share up-to-date and authoritative information that can give readers greater personal control over their health maintenance.

Library of Congress Cataloging-in-Publication Data
Hatfield, Densie, 1953-
Tooth and gum care.
(Health and fitness series)
Includes index.
1. Teeth—Care and hygiene. 2. Gums—Care and hygiene. I. Dudrick, Stanley J. II. American Family Health Institute. Medical Board. III. Title. IV. Series. [DNLM: 1. Dentistry—popular works. 2. Gingival Diseases—popular works. WU 140 H362t]
RK61.H35 1986 617.6'01 86-5725
ISBN 0-87434-029-2

The procedures and explanations given in this publication are based on research and consultation with medical and nursing authorities. To the best of our knowledge, these procedures and explanations reflect currently accepted medical practice; nevertheless, they can't be considered absolute and universal recommendations. For individual application, treatment suggestions must be considered in light of the individual's health, subject to a doctor's specific recommendations. The authors and the publisher disclaim responsibility for any adverse effects resulting directly or indirectly from the suggested procedures, from any undetected errors, or from the reader's misunderstanding of the text.

Contents

Tooth & Gum Care

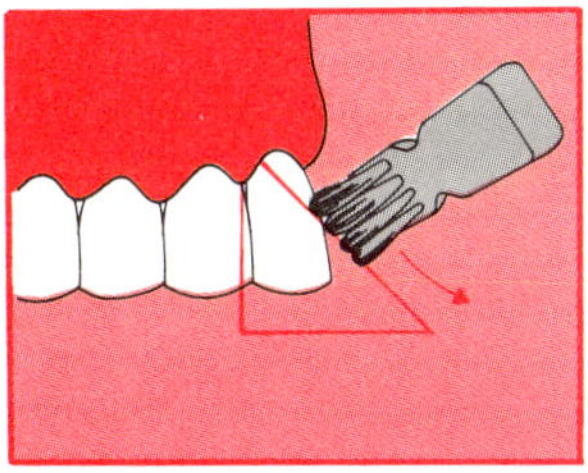

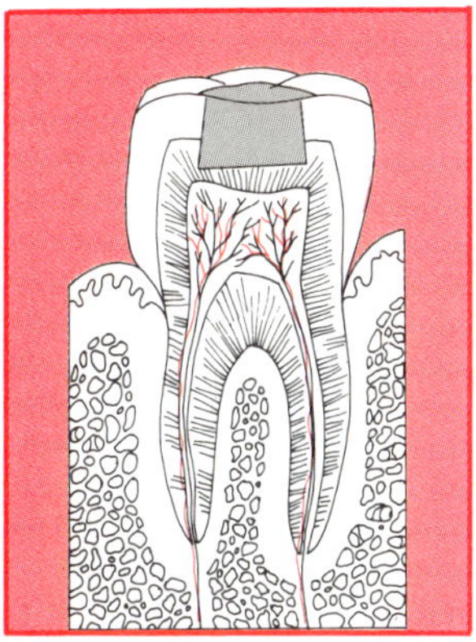

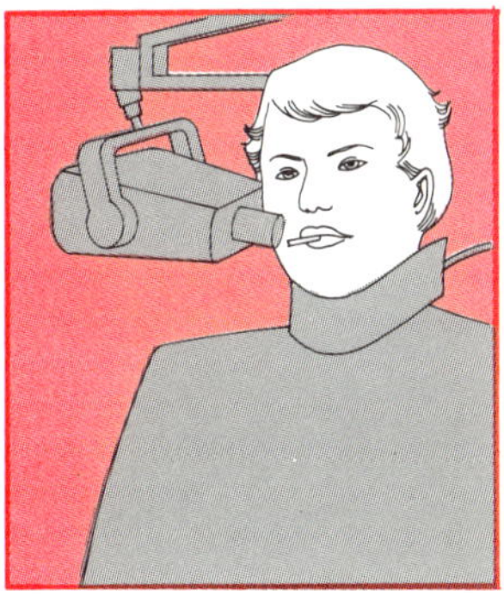

1 Preventing Tooth and Gum Diseases

Prevention is the key to tooth and gum care. You can prevent nearly all dental problems by maintaining good oral hygiene. This means cleansing your teeth both of food particles and of the acid-producing bacteria that live on tooth surfaces and just beneath the gumline.

Maintaining good oral hygiene

Follow these steps to keep your teeth and gums healthy.

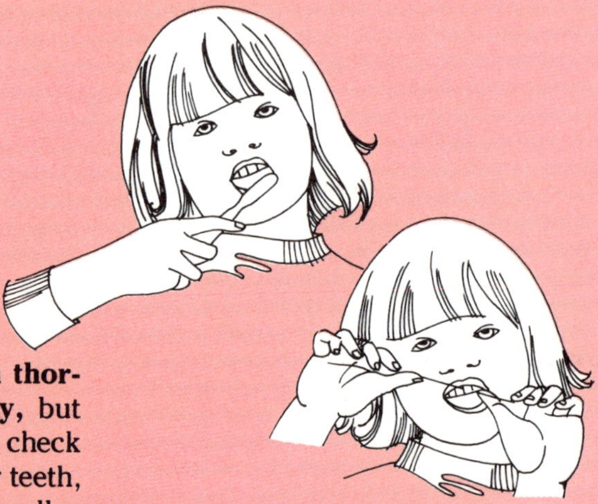

Brush and floss your teeth thoroughly at least once a day, but preferably after each meal. To check how well you're cleaning your teeth, use disclosing tablets occasionally.

Use dental products containing fluoride. Use a toothpaste with fluoride, and ask your dentist about fluoride mouthwashes or rinses.

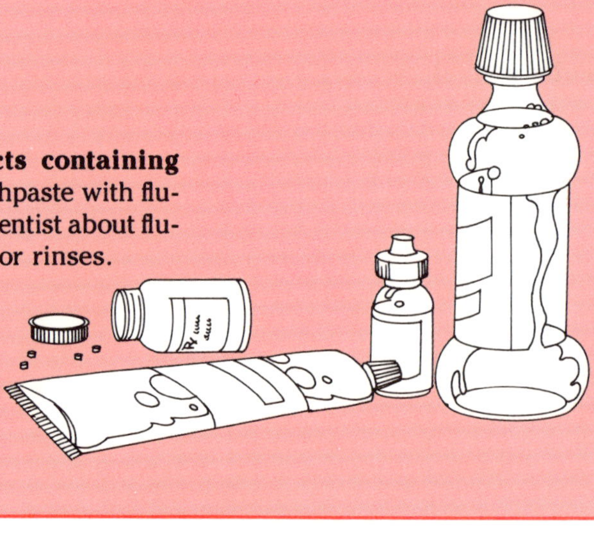

Prevention of tooth decay and gum disease involves these simple practices:

- Brush and floss your teeth thoroughly at least once a day—whenever possible, brush and floss after every meal.
- Use dental products containing fluoride.
- Eat foods that contain starch only with meals, and avoid between-meal snacks.
- Get regular dental checkups.

Prevention of tooth decay and gum disease isn't difficult, and the rewards of prevention are healthy teeth that will last you a lifetime.

Eat starchy and sugary foods with meals only, and avoid between-meal snacks. Candy, sweet snacks, sweet drinks, and dried fruits like raisins are particularly harmful between meals—better to eat your sweets with meals and clean your teeth afterward. Some foods, such as celery and apples, help clean teeth; other foods, such as cheese (especially cheddar), neutralize acid formation.

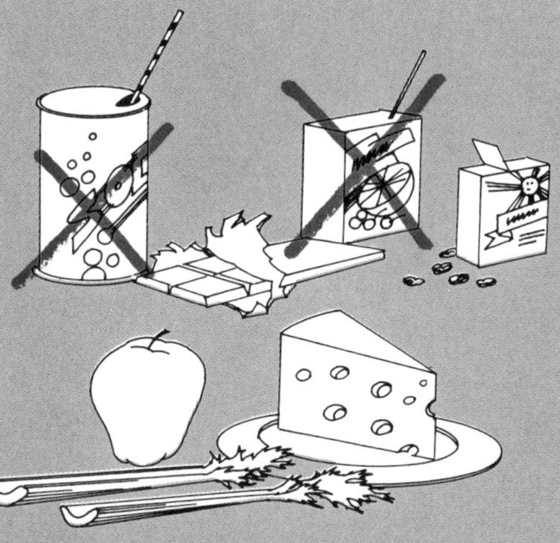

Get regular dental checkups, at least once every 6 months. Such regular checkups ensure that any new cavity is detected and treated before decay can spread and that any developing gum disease is treated before it becomes serious.

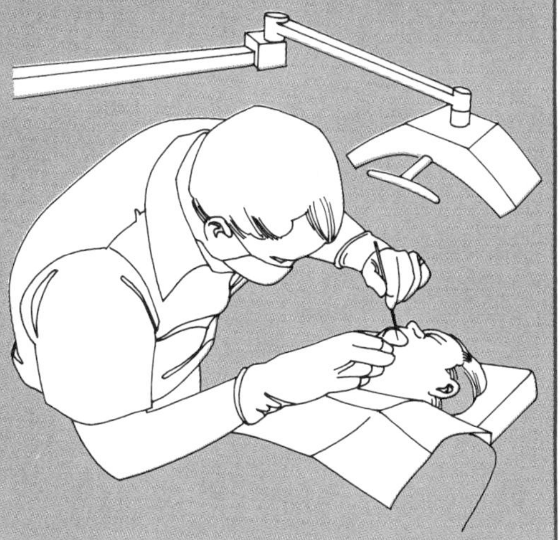

How plaque forms

Most tooth decay and gum disease result from the destructive action of bacteria that live in your mouth. These bacteria live in a gummy film called plaque.

A mixture of bacteria, saliva, mucus, and blood cells from your gums, plaque is constantly forming on your teeth. Plaque sticks to the surfaces of teeth and builds up between teeth and just under the gumline. The bacteria in plaque are most harmful when they become organized into colonies or groups, a process that takes about 24 hours.

Bacteria in the plaque break down carbohydrates (sugars and starches) in your food, and this action produces acid. This acid can wear away a tooth's enamel, eventually forming a tiny cavity—the beginning of tooth decay.

Plaque can also damage gums. If plaque isn't removed daily, it builds up and forms a hard deposit, called tartar, that irritates the gums. Irriated gums may retreat from the tooth's edge, creating a gum pocket where harmful bacteria can gather. Tartar can be removed only with the proper instruments by a dental professional.

The goal of brushing and flossing is the removal of food particles and plaque. By cleaning away food particles, you help control the growth of bacteria; by removing plaque, you protect your teeth and gums from damage.

You can remove plaque from the outer surfaces of your teeth by brushing. The plaque that forms between the teeth and just under the gumline can't be removed by brushing. To remove this plaque, you'll need dental floss.

Brushing and flossing your teeth at least once a day—but preferably after each meal—is the only way to remove food particles and prevent plaque from forming. You can't remove plaque by rinsing your mouth with water or even by just brushing. You must brush and floss.

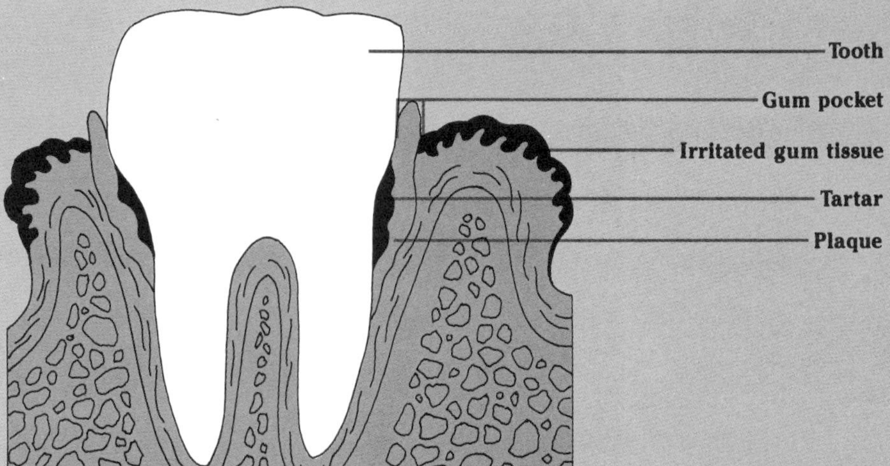

Cavities and the pH of plaque

Plaque causes cavities, and some authorities believe that the acidity or alkalinity (measured as pH) of the plaque on your teeth may determine just how many cavities you'll get. Acidic plaque (pH below 5.5) harms your teeth by dissolving tooth enamel.

Here are some common foods that can cause plaque pH to fall below 5.5.

Apples, dried
Apples, fresh
Apple drink
Apricots, dried
Bananas
Beans, baked
Beans, green, canned
Bread, white
Bread, whole wheat
Caramel
Carrots, cooked
Cereals, non-presweetened
Cereals, presweetened
Chocolate, milk
Cola beverage
Cookies, vanilla sugar
Cornflakes
Cornstarch
Crackers, soda
Cream cheese
Doughnuts, plain
Gelatin dessert, flavored
Grapes
Milk, whole
Milk, 2%
Milk, chocolate
Oatmeal, instant, cooked
Oats, rolled
Oranges
Orange juice
Pasta
Peanut butter
Peas, canned
Potato, boiled
Potato chips
Raisins
Rice, instant, cooked
Sponge cake, cream-filled
Tomato, fresh

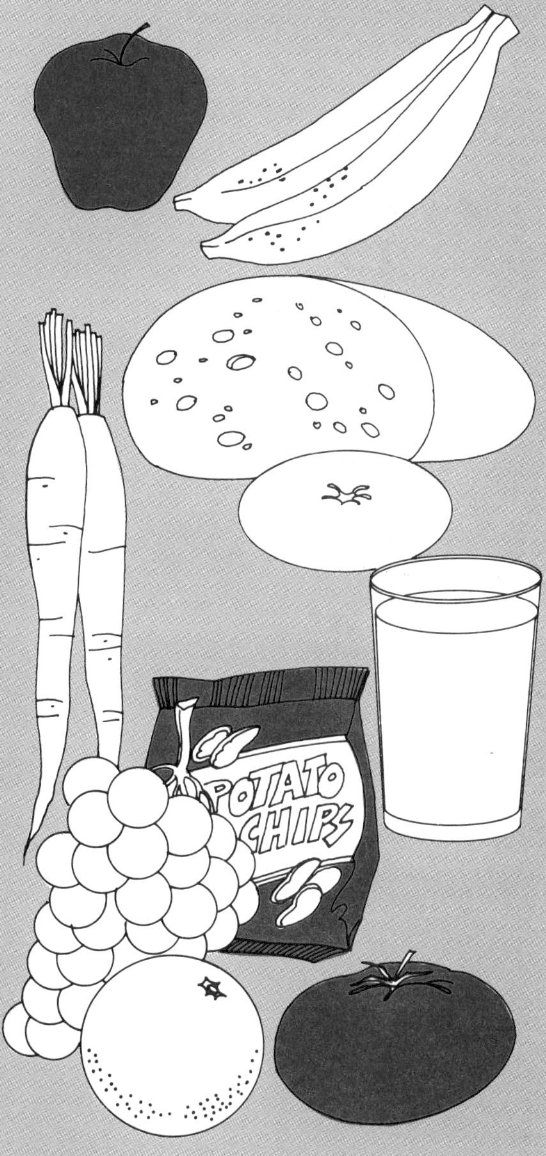

Hard or soft?

Many dentists once recommended that their patients use toothbrushes with hard, natural bristles. However, because natural bristles can cut and irritate gums, most dentists now recommend the use of soft, nylon brushes.

Electric toothbrushes

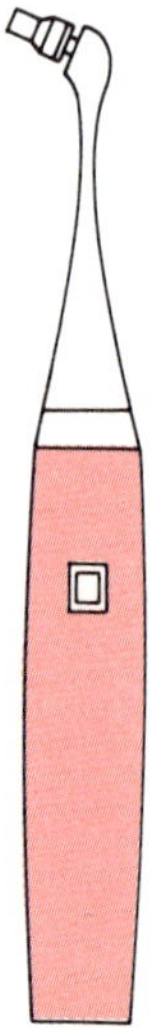

Many people, particularly small children and the handicapped, find maneuvering a toothbrush difficult; an electric toothbrush may be the answer. Used properly, an electric toothbrush can clean teeth as effectively as a nonelectric toothbrush.

Toothbrushes

A good toothbrush is essential to cleaning your teeth properly. The American Dental Association (ADA) recommends the use of a soft, multitufted brush with rounded bristles and a flat brushing surface. The bristles on most soft toothbrushes are made of nylon. These nylon brushes are very effective in removing plaque from teeth without irritating gums.

The head of the toothbrush should be small enough to reach the sides of all your teeth. If you have a small mouth, you may find it easier to use a child's toothbrush.

Replace your toothbrush every 3 to 4 months. If your toothbrush is worn down and the bristles are flattened or pointing in all directions, it won't clean your teeth properly.

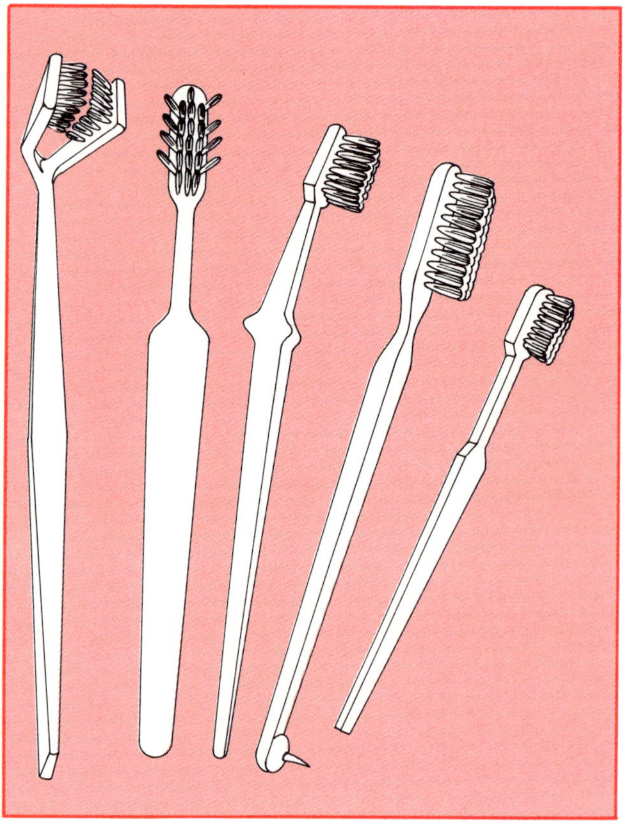

Choosing a toothbrush

Toothbrushes vary extensively. To select one, read the package description and suggested use.

Forgot your toothbrush?

If you find yourself in the unpleasant situation of not having a toothbrush and being unable to buy another right away, you should still clean your teeth. Rinsing your mouth with water doesn't remove plaque but does remove the food particles that promote bacterial growth. If you have toothpaste, you can use your index finger as a substitute toothbrush. Apply some toothpaste to your finger and go over your teeth as best you can. Of course, if you have dental floss, use it. Flossing is every bit as important as brushing. The most important step is to get another toothbrush as soon as possible.

Three times a day

How many times have you been told to "brush three times a day"? And how many times have you actually done it? The "three times" are, of course, after each of the day's three meals, and ideally you should clean your teeth each time you eat. Doing so involves some obvious inconveniences—you can't always have your toothbrush, toothpaste, and dental floss with you. So brush after meals when you can and make sure you clean your teeth thoroughly—using both your toothbrush and dental floss—at least once a day.

Toothpastes

From the many different brands and types of available toothpaste, how do you choose the one that's best for you? First and foremost, look for a toothpaste that contains fluoride. Fluoride reduces tooth decay by hardening tooth enamel, thus protecting teeth from the acids produced by bacteria. Fluoride also prevents bacteria from becoming attached to teeth. However, not all fluoride toothpastes are equally effective in preventing tooth decay. Look for the seal of the American Dental Association Council on Dental Therapeutics on the toothpaste package. Only those toothpastes proven helpful in preventing tooth decay bear this seal.

Several special varieties of toothpaste are now available, including smokers' toothpastes, toothpastes for sensitive teeth, and "anti-plaque" formula toothpastes.

Smokers' toothpastes are designed to help remove the stains that tobacco smoking leaves on teeth. These toothpastes are effective because they're abrasive—they rub away the stains by friction. This rubbing can actually wear down the enamel on teeth, so these toothpastes should be used only once a day.

If your teeth and gums are especially sensitive, you may want to try one of the toothpastes designed for sensitive teeth. But don't depend on one of these toothpastes without checking with your dentist. These toothpastes relieve discomfort but don't cure dental problems. And be forewarned: they aren't as sweet and pleasant tasting as most regular toothpastes.

The newest toothpastes are the so-called anti-plaque formula toothpastes. The American Dental Association is in the process of developing specific guidelines to evaluate the effectiveness of the many new anti-plaque formula toothpastes. To date, none of these toothpastes has received the ADA seal for an ability to fight plaque. Any toothpaste that now carries the ADA seal does so solely because of its fluoride content.

How to brush your teeth

1. Place the toothbrush head with the tips of the bristles angled against the gumline at a 45-degree angle.

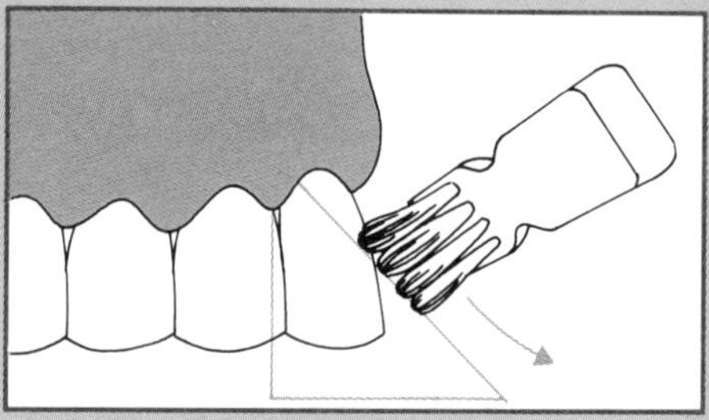

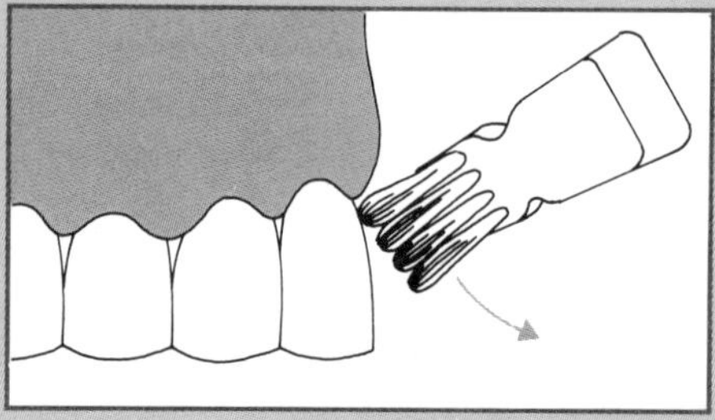

2. Move the brush back and forth with a short (half-a-toothwide) stroke several times. Alternate this motion with curved strokes away from the gumline.

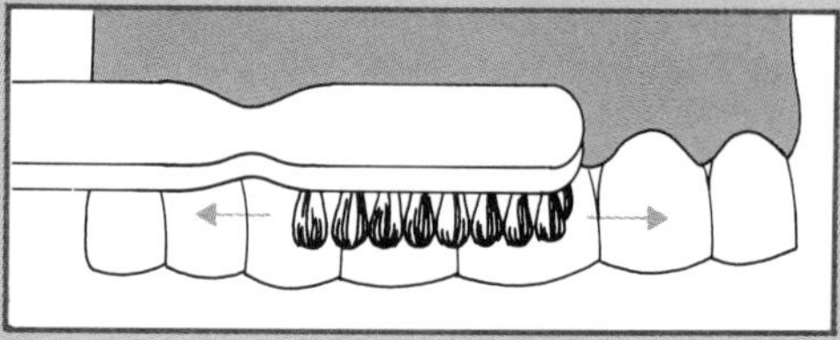

3. Brush the outer surfaces of each tooth, upper and lower, keeping the bristles angled against the tooth.

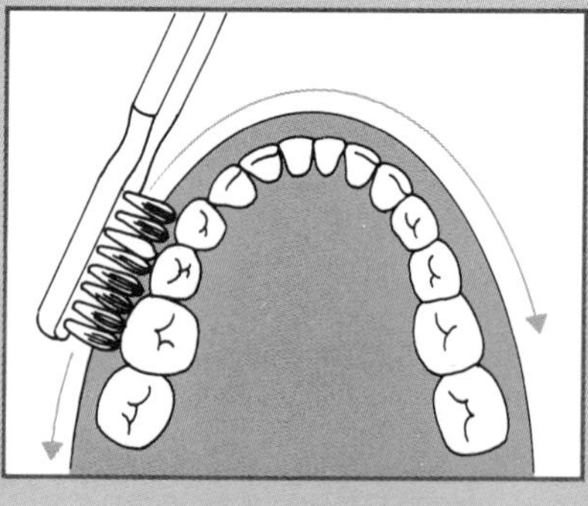

4. Use the same method on all the inside surfaces of your teeth, upper and lower, alternating the short back-and-forth strokes with upward strokes.

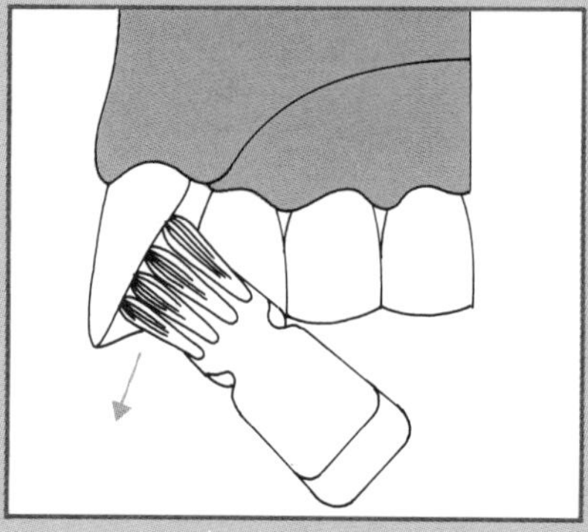

5. Scrub the chewing surfaces of all teeth, upper and lower. Don't press hard; let the bristles get into the grooves of your teeth.

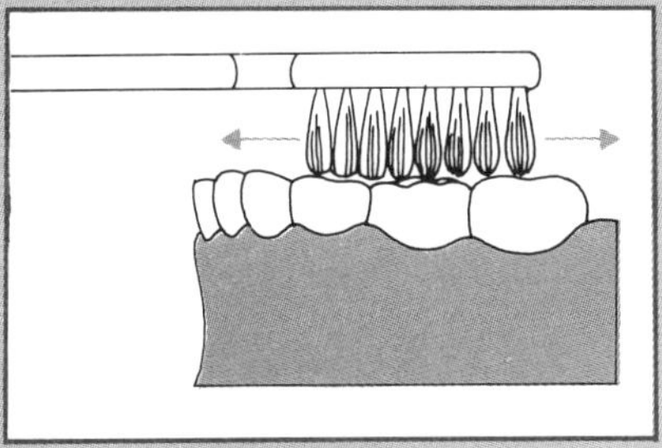

6. Brush the insides of your front teeth by tilting the toothbrush and making several strokes downward (away from gumline) with the tip of the brush.

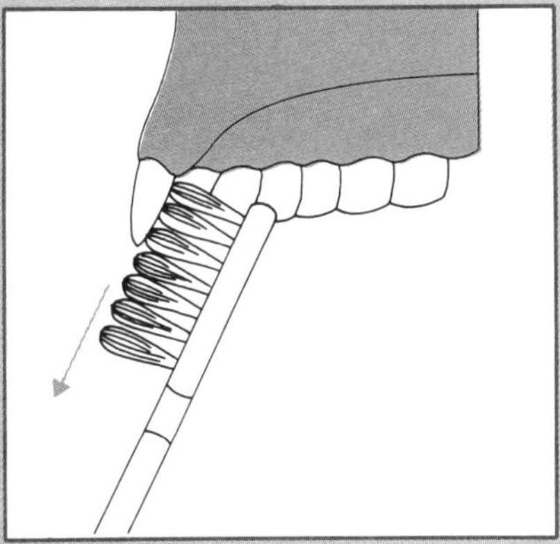

7. Brush your tongue. Bacteria form on your tongue, and brushing your tongue will help freshen your breath.

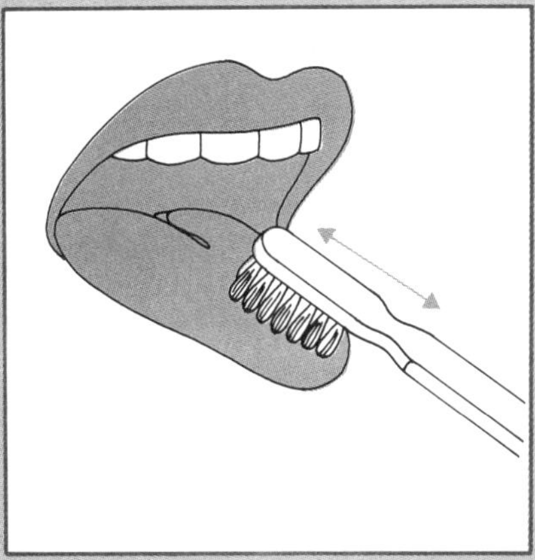

- Always brush gently with very short strokes. Brush just hard enough that you can feel the bristles against your gum.
- Don't squash the toothbrush against your teeth—only the tips of the bristles clean.
- Change the position of the toothbrush frequently as you brush—you should clean only one or two teeth at a time.
- Use a dry toothbrush. You might keep two brushes, alternating them.

Brush and floss or floss and brush?
Which should you do first, brush or floss? Most dentists recommend brushing followed by flossing. Don't forget to rinse your mouth when you've finished flossing—this washes away the loosened food particles and bacteria.

Dental tape
Dental tape, which is wider than dental floss, also removes plaque well. However, if your teeth are very closely spaced, you may experience difficulties maneuvering dental tape between them.

Proper flossing
Ask your dentist or dental hygienist to show you how to use dental floss properly. Incorrect use of dental floss can damage your gums, so take the time to learn the right way.

Homemade toothpaste

Some dentists recommend the use of a homemade toothpaste composed of baking soda, hydrogen peroxide, and salt. The recipe is:

½ teaspoon salt
½ teaspoon baking soda
5 to 6 drops hydrogen peroxide

This mixture makes the inside of your mouth less acidic, which inhibits the growth of bacteria. It doesn't have the pleasant taste of a commercial toothpaste, however, and the hydrogen peroxide will froth a little when it mixes with your saliva. The mixture is also quite salty—if you're watching your sodium intake, take care not to swallow any of the mixture and rinse your mouth well after brushing. If your doctor has you on a sodium-restricted diet, you shouldn't use this mixture. Because the baking soda is somewhat abrasive, you should use this mixture only once a day. Of course, this homemade toothpaste doesn't contain fluoride.

Dental floss

Dental floss is special thread that you pull between your teeth. Flossing—using dental floss—is the best way to remove plaque and food particles from between your teeth and under your gumline, areas your toothbrush can't reach.

Dental floss is available in three varieties: waxed, unwaxed, and partially waxed. Unwaxed dental floss is the most effective in removing plaque because it rubs harder against the smooth surfaces of your teeth. However, you may have difficulty passing unwaxed floss through the tighter areas between your teeth—the floss may break or shred. If you have trouble with unwaxed floss, try the waxed or partially waxed varieties.

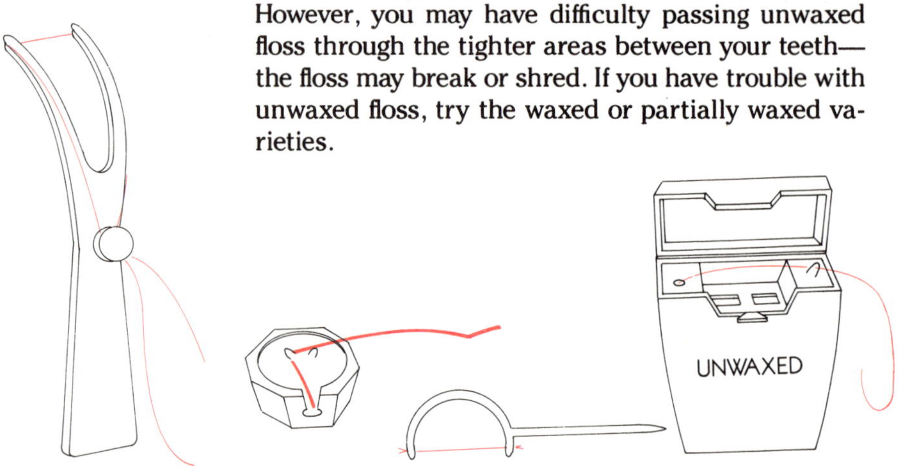

Flossing products, left to right: *floss holder, waxed dental floss, disposable floss holder, unwaxed dental floss*

Toothpicks
Toothpicks aren't a substitute for dental floss. Toothpicks can injure gums if used improperly; or they can break, leaving splinters or tips imbedded between your teeth.

Learning to use dental floss properly takes time and practice. Don't become frustrated if you don't master the technique right away. The complete process may take you 15 or 20 minutes when you first begin; with practice, however, flossing your teeth should take only 5 to 10 minutes.

Oral irrigation devices

Oral irrigation devices use pulsating water sprayed under pressure to remove food particles from hard-to-reach places. These devices are designed to help people with braces or bridgework clean away food particles. Oral irrigation devices are best used by people over age 12.

Two types of oral irrigation devices are available. One uses a motor-driven pump to spray a jet of water; the other is attached directly to a water faucet. Whichever type you use, be careful in the beginning to set the water pressure on low—excessive water pressure can damage your gums. Point the tip of the instrument away from your gumline and work the tip from the gumline to the chewing surface of the tooth. Be careful not to spray food particles back toward the gum—doing so may force the particles under the gum.

Oral irrigation devices *can't* remove plaque and are no substitute for your toothbrush and dental floss. Instructions are provided by the manufacturer, but if you're interested in using an oral irrigation device, you should ask your dentist for further instructions.

A refreshing experience

Oral irrigation devices remove some food particles with the water jet. What's more, you may find the experience refreshing. Just remember that the use of an oral irrigation device can't replace your normal brushing and flossing routine.

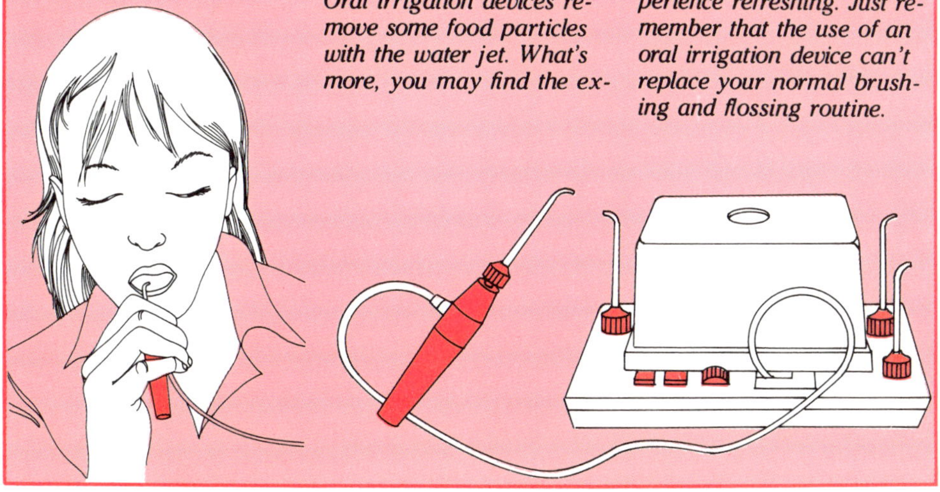

How to use dental floss

1. Take about 18 inches of floss from the dispenser and wrap the ends around your middle fingers, holding a section of about 1½ inches between the thumbs and forefingers.

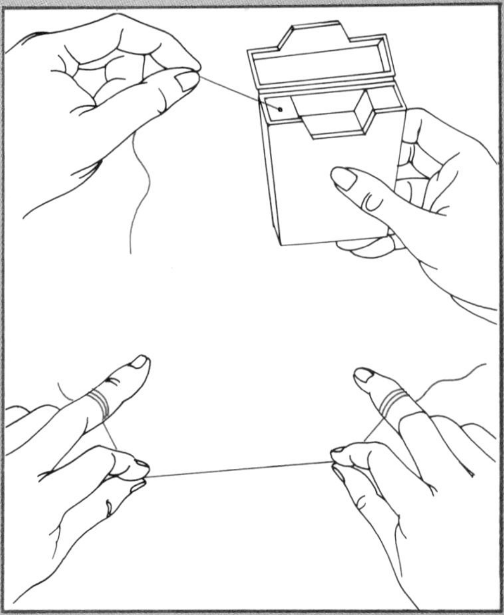

2. Insert the floss between two teeth with a gentle sawing motion; move the floss against and then just beneath the gumline. Be careful: if you force the floss down with one motion, you may cut your gums.

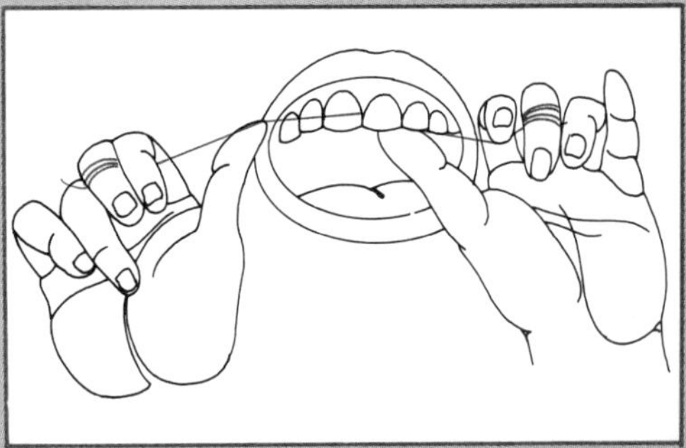

3. Now curve the floss around one tooth into a C shape and slide it into the space between the gum and the tooth until you feel resistance. Then move the floss up and down, gently scraping against the side of the tooth.

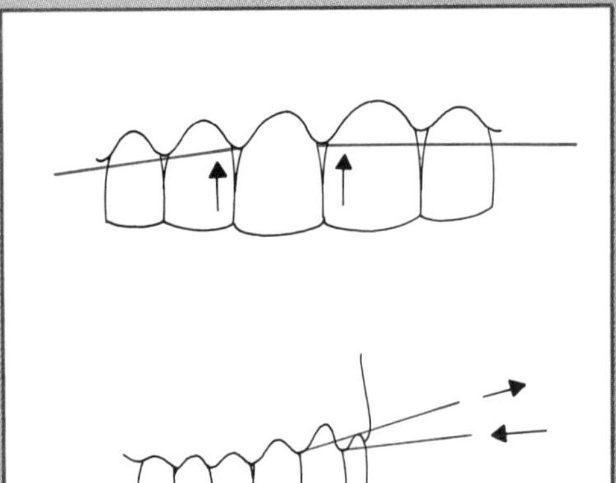

4. Curve the floss around the neighboring tooth and repeat the procedure. Then gently pull the floss out from between these two teeth and move onto the next pair of teeth. Repeat this procedure until you've flossed all your teeth. Don't forget all the sides, including the backside, of your last tooth. Even with proper brushing, plaque can easily build up between your gums and the last tooth.

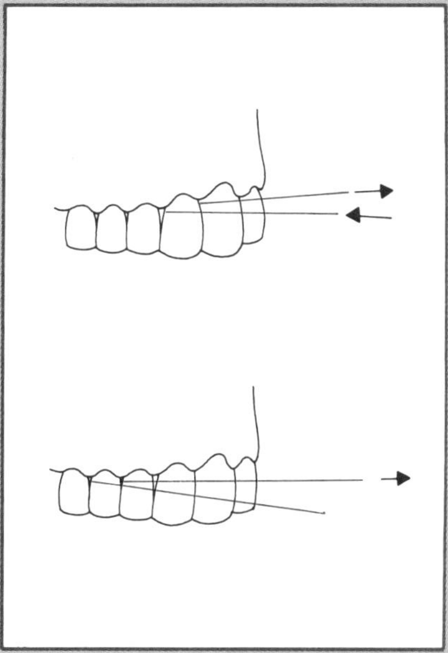

5. Establish a regular time and pattern for flossing so you won't miss any of your teeth on any day. When you've finished flossing all your teeth, rinse your mouth thoroughly to wash out the loosened food particles and bacteria.

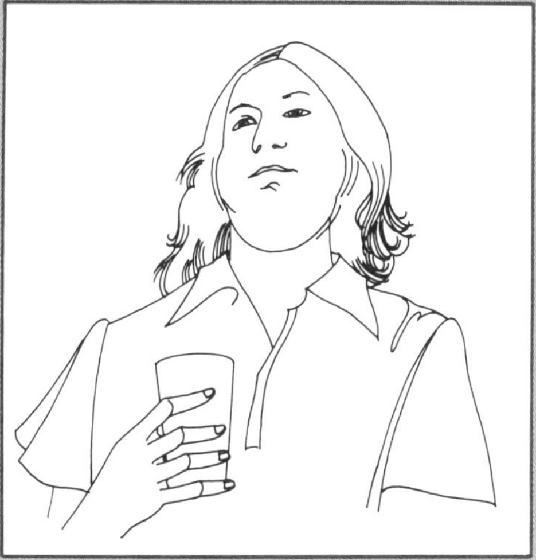

- Your gums may bleed and be sore for the first 5 or 6 days after you start daily flossing. But as you break up plaque and remove bacteria, your gums will heal, and the bleeding will stop. However, if you forget to floss for any length of time and begin again, bleeding may start again. You can avoid this bleeding by being faithful to a regular flossing routine.
- If the initial bleeding doesn't stop after 6 days, consult your dentist. Improper flossing may be injuring your gums, or the bleeding may be a symptom of disease.
- Always be gentle when you insert floss between your teeth and under the gumline.

A red mouth

The dyes used in disclosing tablets and solutions are harmless vegetable dyes. However, these dyes will stain your tongue and lips for several hours, so you may want to use the disclosing agent at bedtime. You can put petroleum jelly on your lips to prevent staining.

Disclosing tablets

Even with your most careful efforts to brush and floss your teeth, you may miss certain areas. A good way to determine if you're cleaning your teeth thoroughly is to use disclosing tablets or solutions. Available at most pharmacies, disclosing tablets contain a vegetable dye that stains plaque or your teeth.

After you've brushed and flossed, use the tablets or solution according to the package directions. In the case of the tablets, this involves chewing one red tablet, sloshing the liquid around in your mouth, spitting out the excess, and then rinsing with water. Don't worry if you swallow a little of the tablet—it's harmless.

Next, examine your teeth in a good light. Use a dental mirror if you have one; a small hand mirror will do. Your entire mouth and tongue will have a pink or red tint. However, the dark red areas on and around your teeth are the areas that you haven't cleaned thoroughly: the dye stains the plaque. You should remove the highlighted plaque. To remove the dye, brush and floss your teeth again, paying special attention to the dark red stains.

At first, you may want to use the disclosing agent every day, but after you learn which areas are giving you difficulties, you'll need to use the disclosing agent only once or twice a week.

Disclosing tablets highlight tooth plaque, helping you clean all surfaces thoroughly.

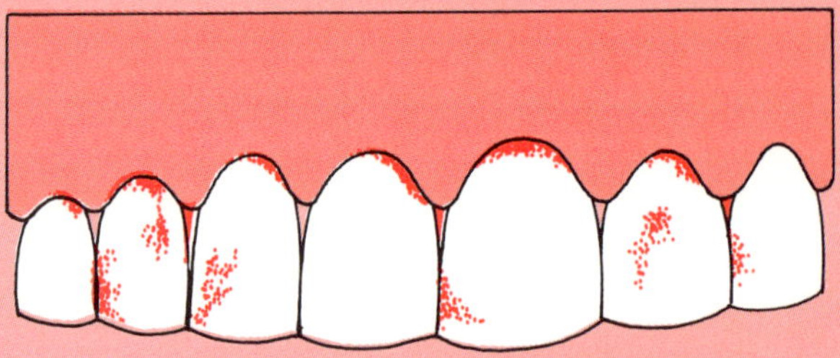

Mouthwashes

Mouthwashes, available in nearly every color, can temporarily freshen your breath, but they can't remove plaque or prevent gum disease. However, mouthwashes that contain fluoride may help protect your teeth from decay (remember to always look for the ADA seal of approval).

You may want to use a mouthwash occasionally to eliminate bad breath. For most people, bad breath is a temporary problem resulting from a dry mouth, and we frequently worry about it more than we should. However, chronic bad breath can be a symptom of tooth decay, gum disease, or some other problem not directly associated with your mouth. Overly zealous use of a mouthwash can cover up a problem that the mouthwash can't cure. If you're unsure, talk to your dentist. Excessive use can also irritate the lining of your mouth.

Fluoride

Fluoride reduces tooth decay by forming mineral crystals in the tooth enamel. These crystals protect teeth from the bacteria's decay-causing acids. Fluoride also keeps bacteria from attaching to teeth.

An essential nutrient that helps our bodies form strong bones and teeth, fluoride is present in many common foods, including fish, tea, and vegetables grown in areas where fluoride is in the water.

Fluoride is naturally present in the water supply of many communities. However, some water supplies don't contain enough fluoride to prevent tooth decay—1 part fluoride per million parts of water is required. Where the level is too low, fluoride may be added to the water. The process of adding fluoride to a community's water supply is called fluoridation. Fluoridation is an inexpensive and proven method to improve a community's dental health. Among the organizations that support fluoridation are the American Dental Association, the American Medical Association, and the American Cancer Society.

Fluoride provides the greatest benefits to children. Fluoride in water is incorporated into the tooth structure as part of the enamel even before permanent teeth appear (erupt). Fluoride benefits adults, too, by inhibiting the root decay that can develop as gums recede with age and by deterring new decay around old fillings.

Homemade mouthwashes

You can make your own mouthwashes, which are cheaper and as effective as commercially available ones. For example, salt rinses made with warm water can help relieve sore or inflamed gums. A hydrogen peroxide rinse made with one part warm water to one part hydrogen peroxide can be an effective antibacterial mouthwash. Don't overuse any mouthwash.

Flouride mouthwashes

No mouthwash has been proven to remove plaque. The mouthwashes that contain fluoride, however, provide the benefits of fluoride—they help protect your teeth from decay. In general, mouthwashes are more cosmetic than therapeutic: they'll sweeten your mouth, but they can't prevent disease.

Children and fluoride

Children who drink fluoridated water from birth have 50% to 65% fewer cavities than children who don't drink fluoridated water. And fluoride's preventive benefits continue as children age.

Is your water fluoridated?

Your dentist, local water authority, or public health department can tell you whether or not your community's water supply is fluoridated. If your water isn't fluoridated, you may want to use some of the special fluoride products now available—check with your dentist. Children can benefit from fluoride through tablets or vitamin-fluoride preparations available by prescription. Fluoride drops are available for infants; children under age 12 should have fluoride applied to their teeth by their dentist every year while their enamel is still forming.

Some community water supplies naturally contain too much fluoride. People living in such communities sometimes have mottled teeth (teeth with white or brown spots). Dentists call this condition fluorosis. Fluorosis, the only known adverse effect of fluoride, can occur where the water supply contains 5 parts of fluoride per million parts of water—not where the water supply contains the recommended 1-part-per-million level.

The ADA recommends that even if the water you drink is fluoridated, you should use a fluoridated toothpaste—and if you use a mouthwash, use one that contains fluoride. Remember to look for the ADA seal of approval.

Flouride sources

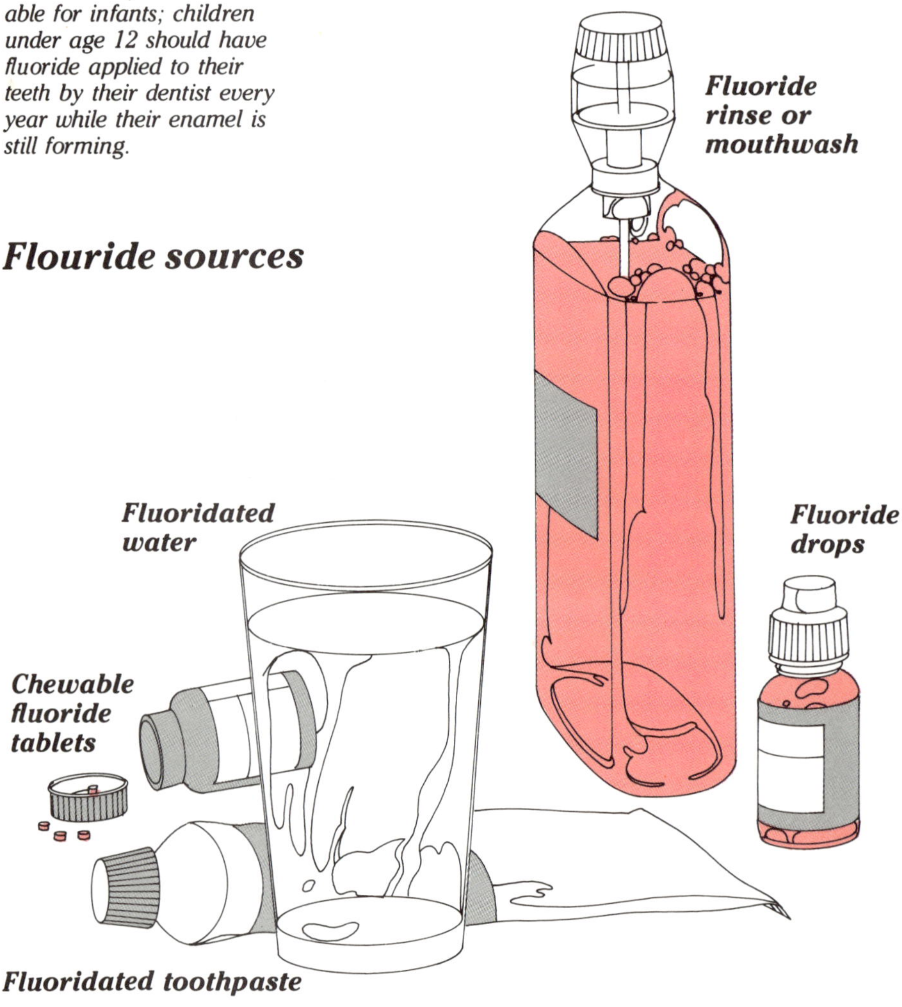

An apple a day

Eating hard, crunchy foods, such as apples, hard rolls, or raw vegetables, can help clean your teeth. Eating such foods also massages your gums and stimulates blood circulation. But don't depend on these foods to clean away sticky food particles left between your teeth. Brushing and flossing are the only way to really clean your teeth.

Nutrition

The food you eat has a direct effect on your dental health. Eating certain foods at the wrong time can promote bacterial growth that results in tooth decay and eventual gum disease.

A diet that's good for the rest of your body will be good for your teeth. Thus, to maintain good dental health, you should eat a balanced diet composed of foods from the basic four food groups.

The basic four food groups

Milk group

Includes milk and everything made from it, such as cheese, ice cream, and yogurt. If you're lowering your fat intake, concentrate on low-fat or skimmed milk, cheeses like cottage cheese and ricotta made from low-fat milk, and yogurt.

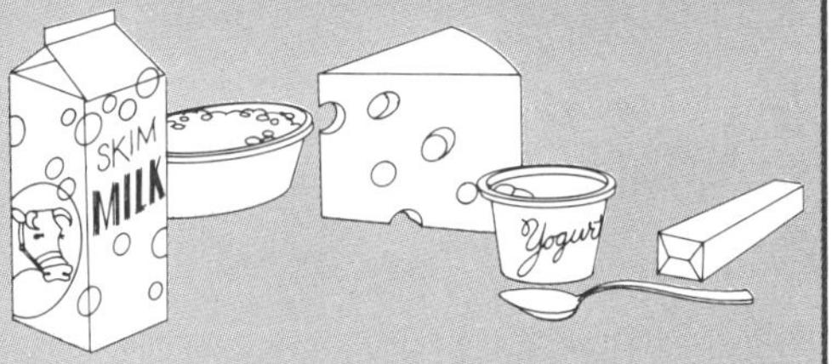

Bread-cereal group

Includes all grains and everything made from them, such as flour and pasta. If you're increasing your intake of fiber, you'll want to eat whole-grain bread and pasta and foods like brown rice, barley, bulgur, millet, and buckwheat.

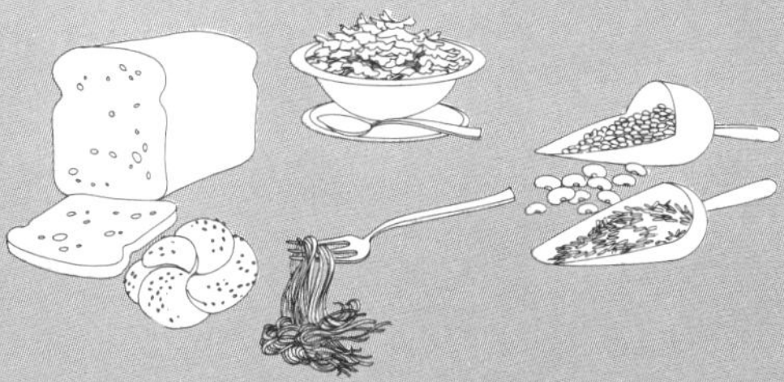

Fruit-vegetable group

Includes all fruits and vegetables. If you're increasing your fiber intake, you'll want to eat a variety of fruits and vegetables. Most are good fiber sources, and some vegetables may contain anticancer factors. Among these are cabbage, kohlrabi, broccoli, cauliflower, and brussels sprouts.

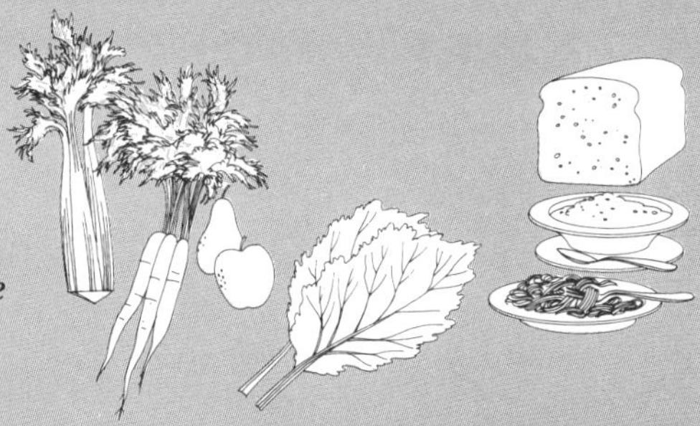

Meat group

Includes beef and other meats, fish, poultry, and eggs. If you're lowering your fat intake, eat more chicken and turkey (remove the skin), rabbit, and fish.

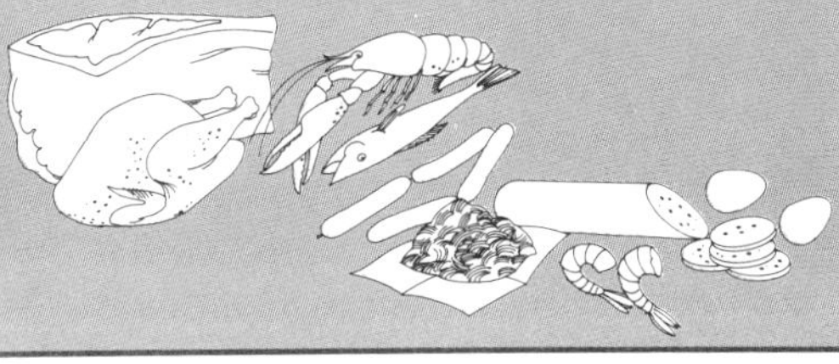

Vitamin C
Vitamin C is necessary for healthy gums. However, vitamin C is an acid (ascorbic acid) and can damage teeth if overused. Taken too often, chewable vitamin C tablets may damage tooth enamel.

Most of the foods harmful to dental health fall into a fifth group composed of the sweet "goodies" we sometimes eat between meals. Examples of these foods are cookies, cakes, candies, pastries, jams, and syrups. A healthy diet limits the amount of such foods, and you've probably already heard that sugary foods are bad for your teeth.

Why is sugar bad for your teeth? Bacteria in your mouth use it to produce acid—the acid that erodes tooth enamel, leading to tooth decay. The bacteria also change starches into sugar, so starchy foods such as crackers, cereals, or pasta can also contribute to tooth decay. The amount of starchy and sugary foods you eat isn't as important as how often you eat such foods, when you eat them, the length of time the foods stay in your mouth (how long you wait before cleaning your teeth), and the foods' form—in particular, how sticky they are. In fact, such foods eaten as part of meals contribute little to tooth decay; but sweet or starchy snacks eaten between meals can lead to decay.

The foods most damaging to teeth are sticky sweets, such as caramels, dried fruits (including raisins), cookies, and pastries. You may be surprised to find raisins on the don't-eat-between-meals list. But raisins are sticky and sweet. Be cautious, too, of so-called health foods or "natural" foods. While such foods may be nutritious and tasty, they may also contain honey, molasses, dates, raisins, and other ingredients that aren't good for your teeth. In terms of your teeth, honey—which sticks to teeth—is worse than refined sugar.

If you don't want to eliminate sweet foods from your diet, make sure you brush—or at least rinse your mouth to remove food particles—after every meal. And avoid between-meal snacks. Better still, cut out sweets altogether. In place of a sugary dessert, you can eat fruit or cheese. Cheese is a particularly good choice because it neutralizes acid formation in your mouth.

Sugar alert

One of the best ways you can guard against cavities is to avoid or at least restrict your consumption of sugary foods that stick to your teeth. Some foods are obviously high in sugar—jam, candy, nondiet soft drinks—but other heavily sugared foods aren't as well known. Here are some of the worst culprits, along with some low-sugar foods for comparison.

Food	Serving size	Teaspoons of sugar per serving
Beverages		
Frozen concentrate imitation orange juice	6 oz	5.4
Sprite	12 oz	9
Coke	12 oz	9.2
Grape juice	6 oz	1
Cereals		
Sugar Smacks	1 cup	16
Cap'n Crunch	1 cup	12
All-Bran	1 cup	3
Shredded Wheat	1 biscuit	0
Condiments		
French salad dressing	1 tbsp	0.7
Italian salad dressing	1 tbsp	0.2
Cranberry sauce	½ cup	11.7
Catsup	1 tbsp	0.6
Other foods		
Vanilla ice cream	½ cup	3.1
Lowfat flavored yogurt	½ cup	4.1
Whole-milk yogurt, fruit	½ cup	7.5
Applesauce	½ cup	4.3
Canned pears or pineapple in heavy syrup	½ cup	3.1
Jello, cherry	½ cup	4.5

Dental X-rays

The most common type of dental X-ray is the bite-wing examination. This view allows your dentist to see the crowns of your teeth, to detect decay between your teeth, and to check the condition of the supporting bone. Bite-wings are usually taken during regular checkups and make use of a small piece of X-ray film covered with a protective casing that you grip firmly between your teeth. Your dentist may cover your torso with a special lead apron or place a lead shield around your neck (to protect your thyroid, which is especially sensitive to radiation).

Another type of dental X-ray is the full-mouth series, which a dentist will take for information on all your teeth, their roots, and the supporting bones. When you see a dentist for the first time, he'll need to take a full-mouth series to provide a record of your dental condition, unless your X-rays are available from another dentist.

Panoramic X-rays show all the teeth and surrounding bone on one large piece of X-ray film. A special X-ray machine is necessary for this procedure. This type of X-ray is useful in examining the growth and development of children's teeth and jaws.

Orthodontists sometimes use cephalometric X-rays, which show a side view of the head, giving the dentist a view of the relationship between the teeth and the skull. Orthodontic treatments can take several years, so the dentist needs to see the changes caused by the growth of the teeth.

Bite-wing X-ray unit

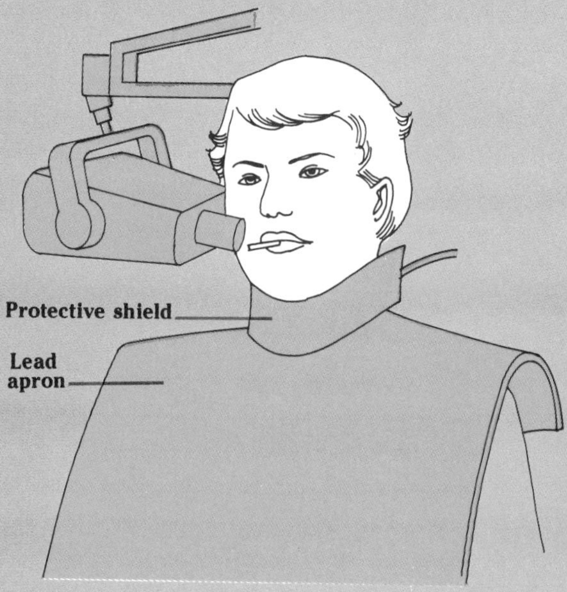

X-ray machine

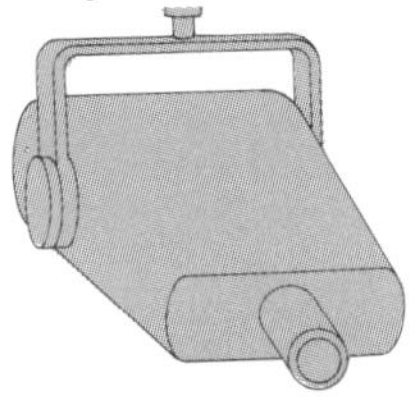

X-ray film and protective casing

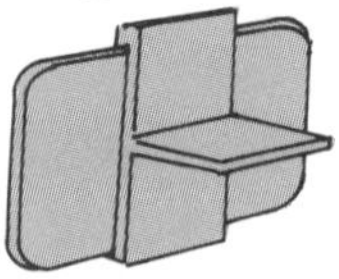

Panoramic X-ray unit

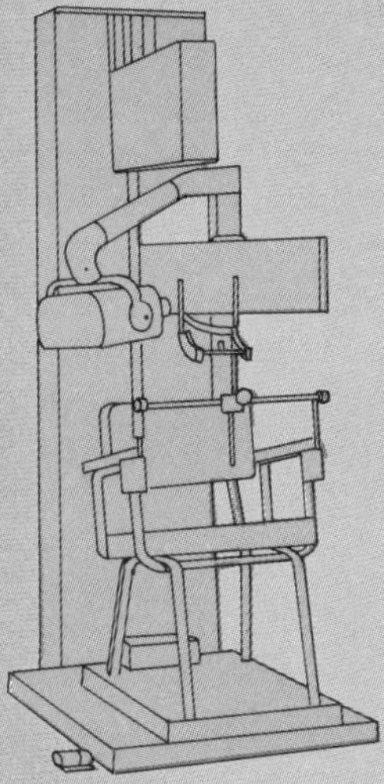

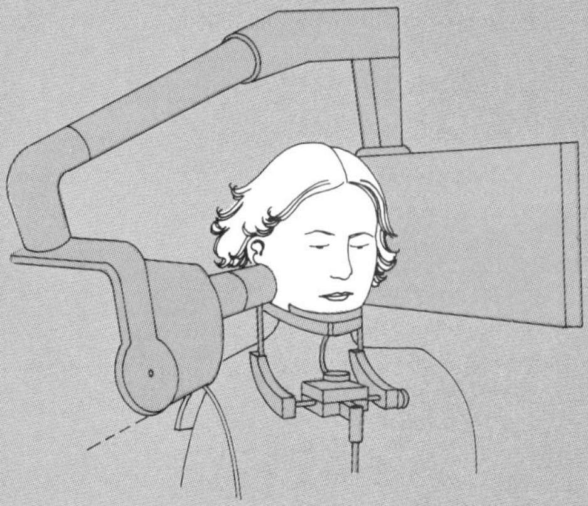

Cephalometric X-ray unit

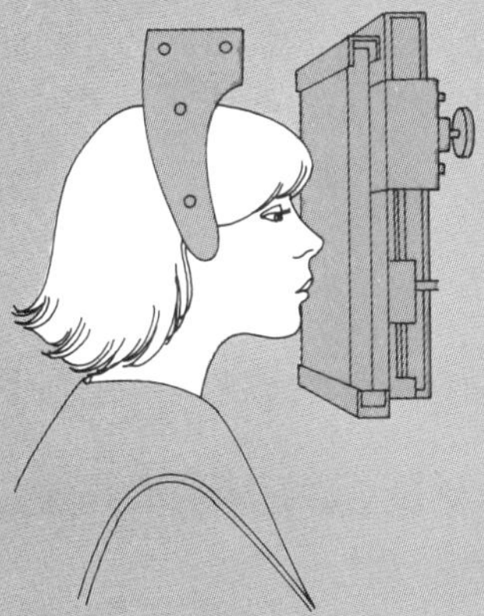

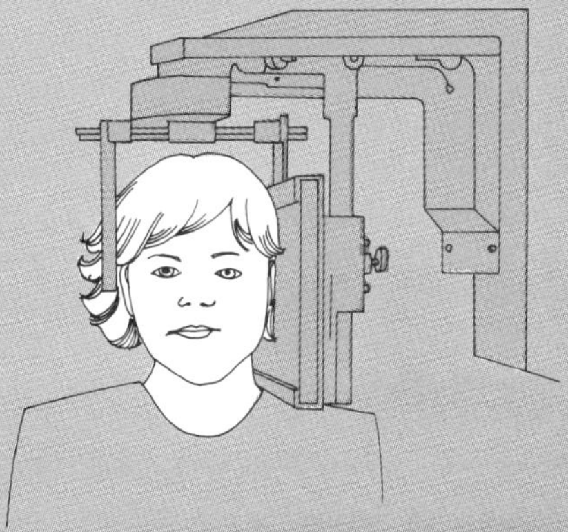

Avoid unnecessary X-rays

Like other X-rays, dental X-rays involve radiation that may increase your risk of cancer. To avoid unnecessary X-rays:

- Ask your dentist why an X-ray is needed. Ask him to take as few as possible.
- Don't insist on X-rays if your dentist explains that they're not required.
- If you change dentists, have your X-ray films sent to your new dentist. That way, you'll avoid another full-mouth series.
- Keep a record of your dental X-rays if you're seeing different dentists at the same time. That way, you can help the dentist determine which X-rays you don't need reshot.

How to find a dentist

If you don't already have a dentist, ask friends, relatives, or co-workers if they can recommend one to you. Or ask your doctor or local pharmacist for a recommendation. Other ways to find a dentist include the following:

- *Check with the dental clinic at a nearby hospital.*
- *Call a nearby dental school and ask for the names of members who have private practices.*
- *Contact the Academy of General Dentistry, 211 East Chicago Avenue, Chicago, Illinois 60611 (312-440-4300), and ask for a list of members in your neighborhood. Members of the academy must maintain high standards.*

Regular dental checkups

See your dentist regularly. Most dentists recommend an examination and cleaning every 6 months. These regular visits ensure that any new cavity will be filled before the decay can spread and that any gum disease will be treated before it can become serious.

During your regular checkups, your dentist will examine your teeth for early signs of decay and your gums and mouth for signs of infection or other problems. Your dentist will then check any fillings you may have to see if any parts have been chipped off or if new cavities are developing around the edge of a filling. Then either your dentist or a dental hygienist will remove the plaque and tartar from your teeth. Every year or two your dentist may take X-rays of your teeth to check for dental problems that can't be detected during the normal checkup.

Be sure to ask your dentist any specific questions you may have about preventive dental care and the oral hygiene procedures you should be doing at home.

Questions to ask your dentist

You may always have a mouthful of questions for your dentist, or you may be the type that prefers to suffer in silence. Either way, you should always ask certain questions before giving the go-ahead for anything but a routine procedure:

- What exactly does this procedure involve—what are you going to do?
- Is this procedure absolutely necessary? Should I get a second opinion?
- How much will this procedure cost? Will my insurance cover it? All of it? If not, how much of it?
- Will the procedure hurt? How much? For how long?
- What type of anesthetic will you give me? What are its possible side effects?

Checking for cavities

During your regular dental visit, your dentist will inspect your teeth with a mirror and a needle-shaped probe. He'll look for any color changes that might indicate decay or any cracks that might indicate the beginning of a cavity. He'll also check your fillings to see if parts have been chipped off or if new cavities are developing around the edges of old fillings.

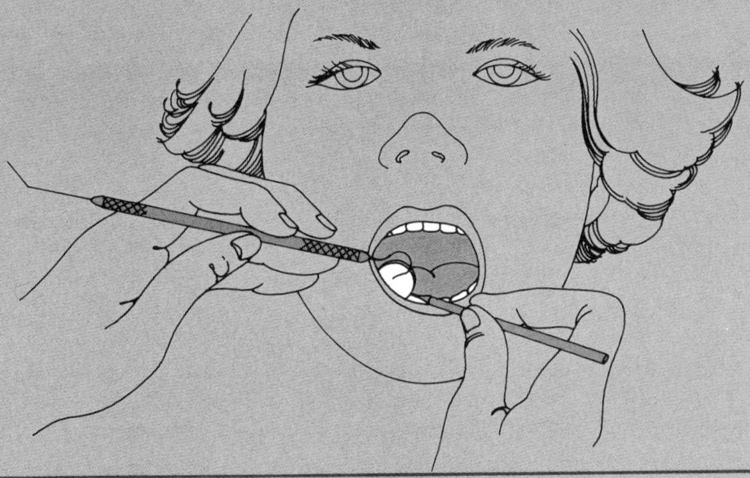

Cleaning and polishing

Your dentist or dental hygienist may use a variety of instruments to remove built-up tartar (calculus): probelike instruments, ultrasonic units, or scalers.

Having removed any tartar, your dentist or dental hygienist will polish your teeth with a special brush. Smooth tooth surfaces retard the growth of plaque and the deposit of new tartar.

Removing tooth tartar

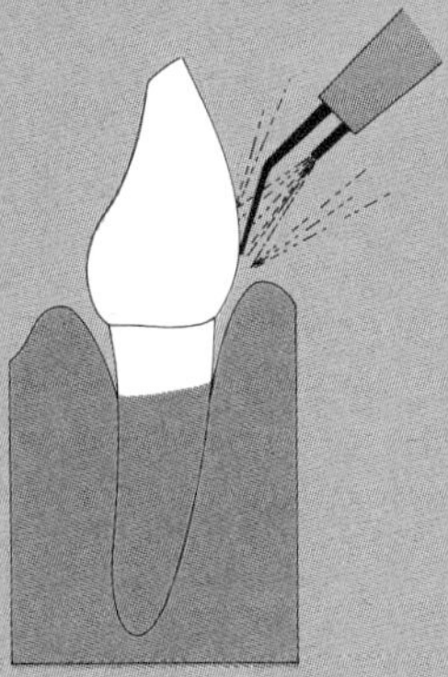

Polishing tooth's surface

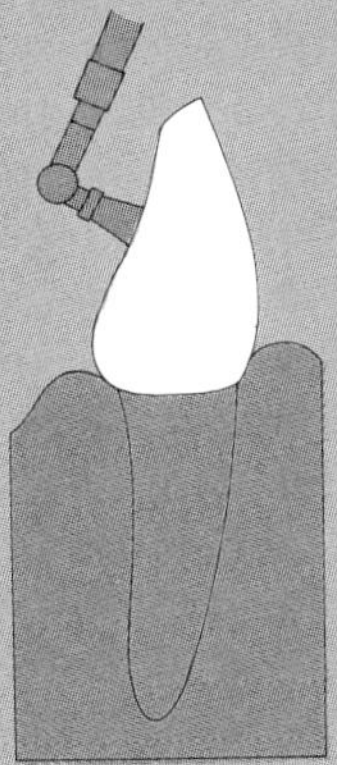

2 Caring for a Child's Teeth

Care of baby teeth
Because children lose their primary teeth, many parents take the attitude that oral hygiene isn't important. However, decay in a primary tooth can lead to decay of the permanent tooth that replaces it. Furthermore, children should be taught good oral hygiene practices early.

At birth, a baby usually has a full set of 20 teeth below the gums, waiting to erupt. These first teeth—known as primary, baby, or "milk" teeth—begin to erupt during the first months and continue to appear and develop for 2 or 3 years. By the time a child is between ages 6 and 8, primary teeth begin to fall out and are replaced by permanent teeth. Between the ages of 6 and 12, most children have a combination of primary and permanent teeth.

Average ages for teeth to appear

These charts outline the average ages at which primary and permanent teeth appear. Remember, the ages given are averages. Early or late teething has no effect on a child's general health. Sometimes not all 20 primary teeth erupt, and sometimes an extra, or supernumerary ("beyond the standard number"), tooth appears. Such extra teeth usually appear between the two front teeth. Thus, a child may have an odd number of teeth.

Primary teeth (usually 20 teeth): Age and order of arrival

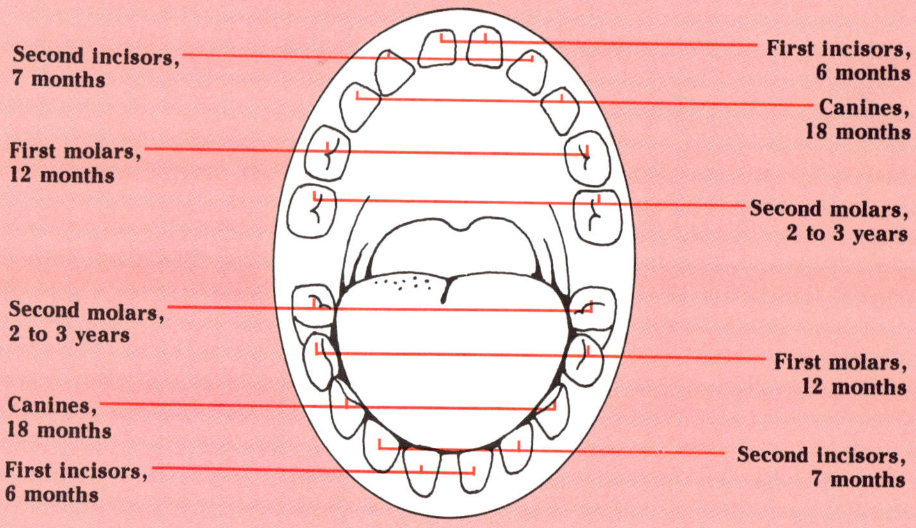

Permanent teeth (usually 32 teeth): Age and order of arrival

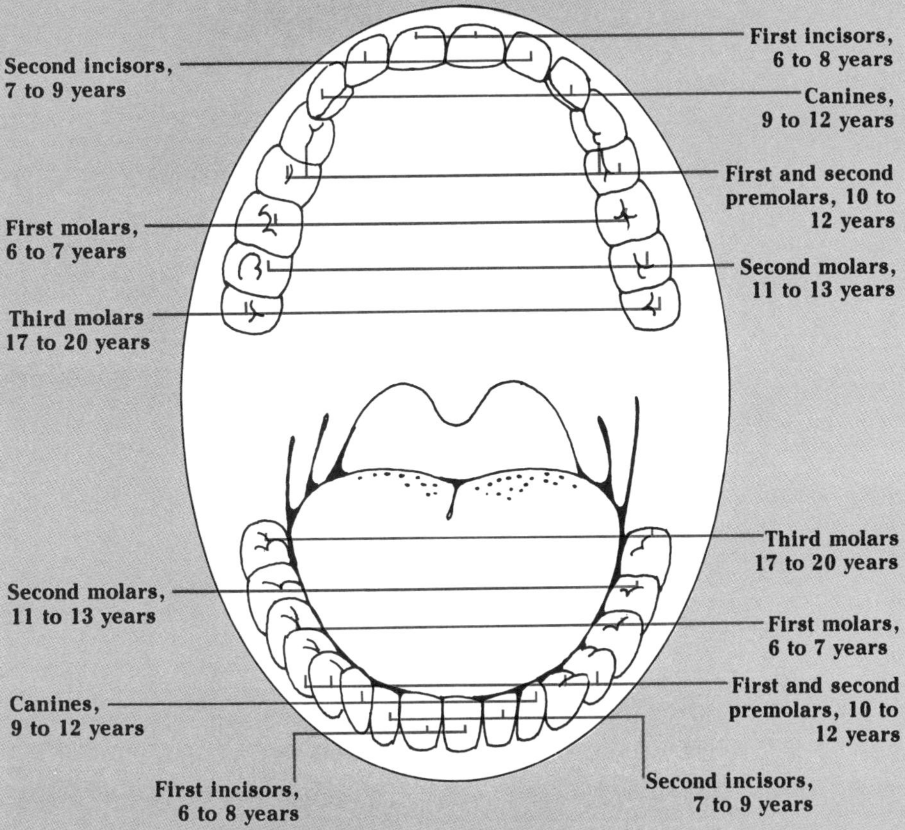

White teeth

The color of your teeth is a reflection of the dentin beneath the enamel. The thinner the enamel, the darker the tooth; the thicker the enamel, the whiter the tooth.

Tooth structure

Each tooth can be divided into two major sections: the crown and the root. The crown is above the gum; the root, buried in the gum, fits into a socket in the jawbone.

If you look at a cross-section of a tooth, you can see that each tooth is composed of overlapping layers. At the center of the tooth is the pulp, which contains blood vessels and nerves that sense heat, cold, pressure, and pain. Around the pulp is a hard substance, called dentin, that forms the bulk of the tooth. Although hard, dentin provides the elasticity necessary to chew hard foods. The dentin receives nutrients from the pulp and can reproduce itself as long as the pulp is healthy.

The dentin is surrounded by a bonelike structure called cementum. Cementum acts as protection around the root portion of the dentin. Around the cementum is connective tissue, known as the periodontal ligament, connecting the root of the tooth to the bone socket.

Tooth structure and shape

This cross-section of a premolar, seen in relation to the surrounding gum, shows the tooth's parts.

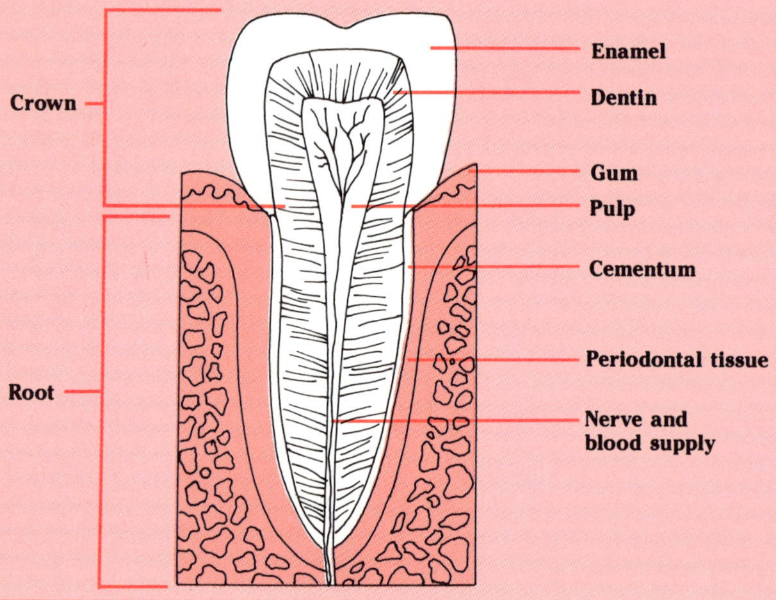

Bedtime bottles
Don't give an infant a bottle of sugar milk or juice to go to bed with as a pacifier. The fluids can gather near the infant's front teeth and cause tooth decay by the time the child is age 3 or 4. If you must give your child a bottle at bedtime, make it a bottle of fluoridated water.

The crown is composed of dentin covered by enamel. This tooth enamel is the hardest substance in your body. It protects and insulates the dentin. Unlike some other body tissues, enamel can't repair itself once it's damaged. Tooth decay begins when acids produced by bacteria erode the enamel.

Basic care

Even before your baby's first tooth erupts (comes through the gum), you can begin protecting your baby's teeth from decay. Use a piece of gauze or a clean washcloth to remove decay-causing bacteria from your baby's mouth. Wipe the gauze or cloth along the gum pads, the ridges where the teeth will appear. Continue this cleaning procedure as your baby's teeth begin to erupt.

Baby teeth must be cared for because decay in a primary tooth can lead to decay of the permanent tooth that replaces it. The most important factors affecting the health of your child's teeth are fluoride, diet, and oral hygiene.

Functions

Teeth cut and grind food, breaking it into pieces that can be easily swallowed and digested. The shapes of teeth differ according to function: incisors and canines are sharp for cutting, whereas molars and premolars are flatter for grinding.

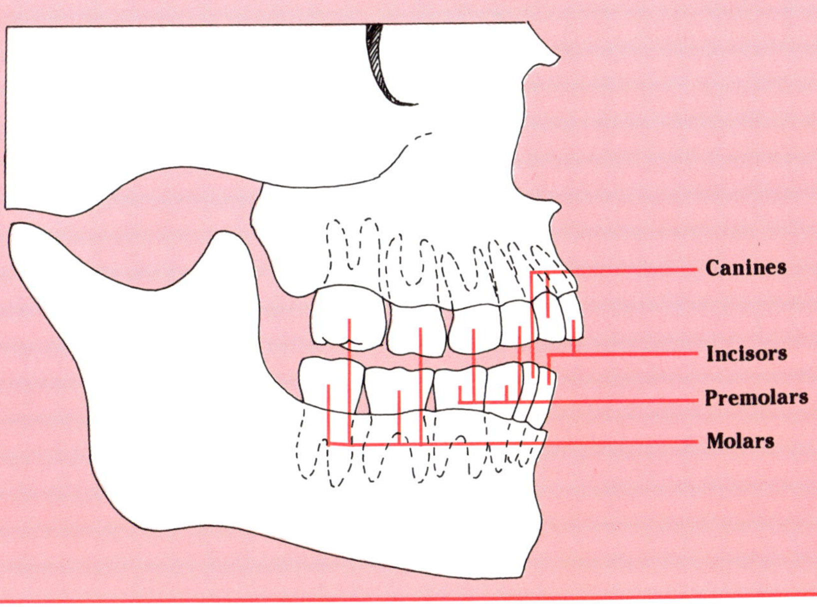

Loose baby tooth?
If your child has a loose baby (primary) tooth that makes chewing difficult and irritates the gums, go ahead and pull it out. A loose tooth pushes against the soft gum tissues, making them sore and inflamed.

Grab the tooth with your fingers or a piece of gauze and give a quick pull. After you've pulled the tooth, press gauze against the gum for a few minutes to stop any bleeding.

If a primary tooth comes out and your child swallows it, don't worry. A tooth is very small and will pass through the child's digestive tract without causing any problems.

Breast milk contains very little fluoride, so if you're breast-feeding your baby, you should add a daily bottle of fluoridated water to your baby's diet. If your community's water supply isn't fluoridated, ask your dentist about fluoride supplements, such as tablets or vitamin-fluoride preparations. Some dentists recommend fluoride drops for infants, and children under age 12 should have fluoride applied to their teeth. During the child's regular checkup, your dentist will fill a mold with fluoride and place it over the child's teeth. The fluoride remains in contact with the teeth for a few minutes.

You can begin flossing your child's teeth by the time he or she is age 3. By age 2, your child should be learning how to handle a toothbrush, and by age 4 or 5 he or she may be able to handle the toothbrush adequately. However, don't let a child under age 7 or 8 brush without supervision. Young children don't have well-developed coordination, so their brushing

Helping your child brush

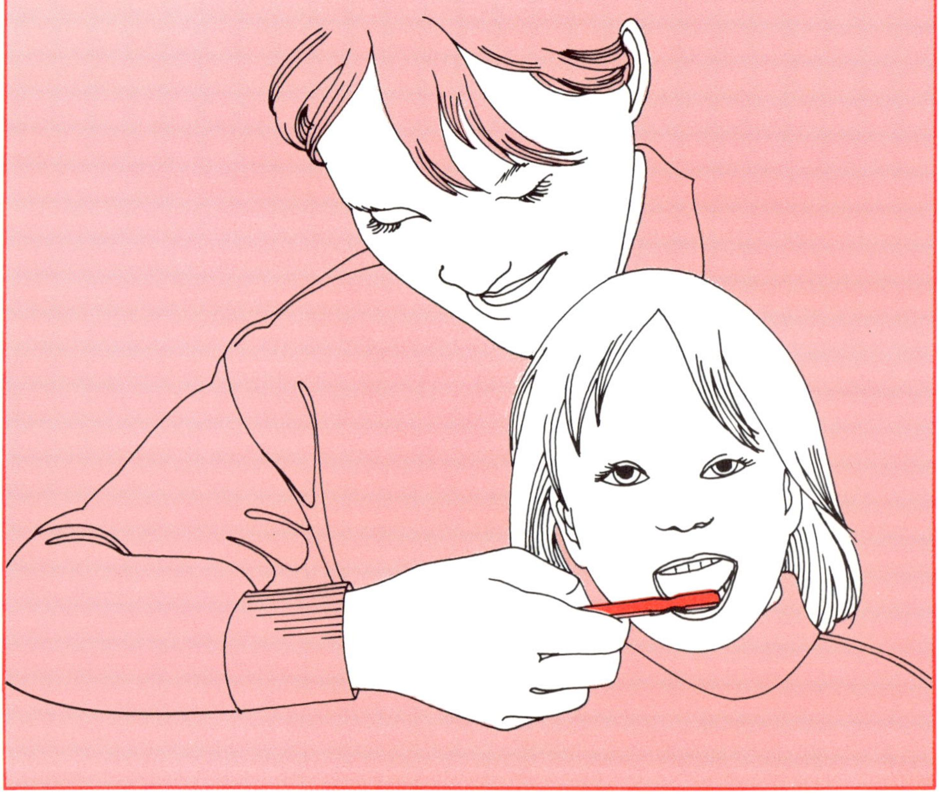

Lemons

Don't let children suck on lemons; lemon juice can destroy tooth enamel.

Brushing fun

An electric toothbrush may inspire your child to brush longer and more carefully. Make certain, however, that your child is brushing his or her teeth and not using the brush as a toy.

technique is likely to be sloppy. What's more, unsupervised young children rarely brush their teeth for longer than 30 seconds.

Get your child a toothbrush with soft, rounded bristles. A special children's toothbrush is best; you'll find a wide range of children's toothbrushes available, beginning with trainer toothbrushes designed for children as young as 7 months. Children's toothbrushes are specially designed for small mouths and small hands and help a child gradually learn how to use a toothbrush. A simple back-and-forth scrubbing motion is usually easier for a child to learn than the alternating motion recommended for adults.

Some children have a great deal of difficulty learning to floss. Lack of coordination is the problem, and your child will outgrow it. To help your child learn to floss, take about 10 inches of floss and tie the ends together. This floss loop is easier to hold than loose ends. Watch your child to make sure he or she uses the floss properly and doesn't injure the gums.

Helping your child floss

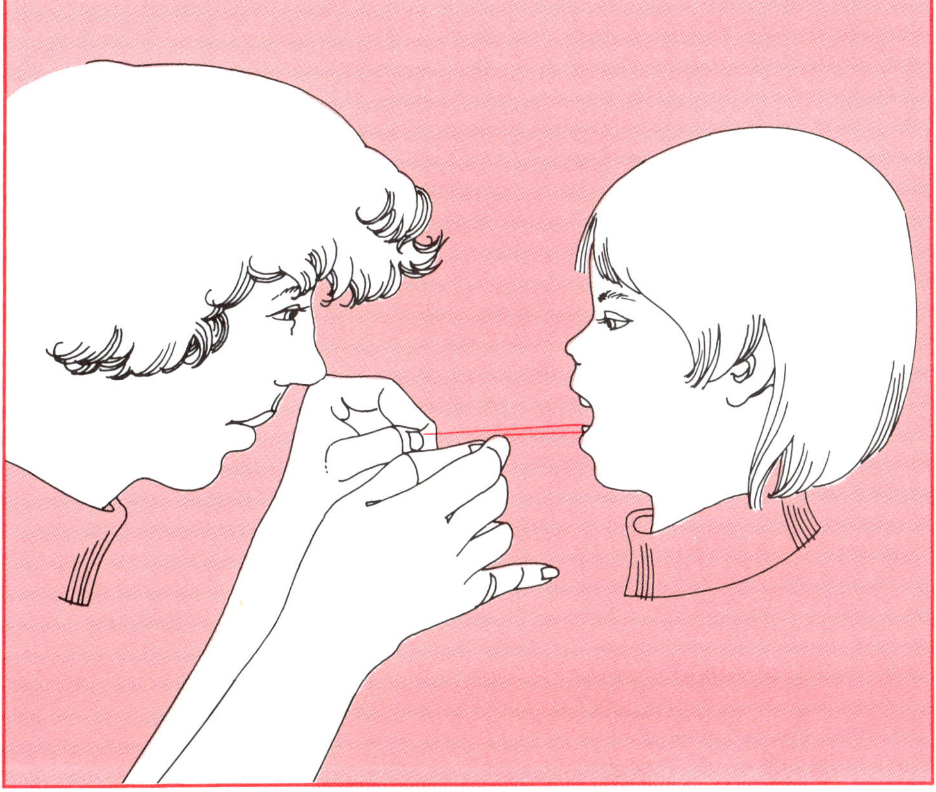

3 Treating Tooth Decay

The symptoms of tooth decay
The first symptom of tooth decay is a mild toothache when you eat something sweet, hot, or cold. If the decay continues, you may have an unpleasant taste in your mouth—the result of food and bacteria stuck in the cavity. If the tooth's pulp becomes inflamed, you may suffer even greater pain when eating sweet, hot, or cold food. You may also experience sharp pain in your jaw above and below the tooth.

Who gets tooth decay?
Only about 2% of the American population never gets cavities. Boys, girls, men, and women are affected equally. Some people seem to be resistant to tooth decay; no matter how badly they neglect their teeth, they don't get cavities. Others seem to be prone to tooth decay and get cavities no matter how often they clean their teeth. Most of us, however, fall somewhere between and can greatly benefit from good oral hygiene practices.

A cavity is a hole in a tooth caused by acid-producing bacteria in plaque. The bacteria break down the carbohydrates in foods left in your mouth; this process produces an acid that can erode tooth enamel. As the acids repeatedly attack the enamel, a small hole develops—a cavity. Left untreated, the decay will spread through the tooth's several layers: the acids will break through the enamel to the dentin. This is when the pain begins. You're most likely to feel the pain when you eat something sweet, very hot, or very cold. If left untreated, the decay will spread to the pulp. The pulp is the "life" of the tooth, providing nourishment to the dentin. When decay reaches the pulp, the pulp may become infected and inflamed. Pus may form in the tissue around the tooth's root: this is called an abscess. An untreated abscess may spread into the jawbone and erode a small canal, or sinus, through the bone and the gum. Before breaking through the gum, the infection will form a swelling, or pocket. This swelling may remain several weeks; sometimes, however, the swelling bursts, draining pus into the mouth. In such cases the pain will suddenly stop; the abscess may appear to have healed. In reality, what may have happened is that the pulp—and the tooth—has died.

Causes of tooth decay

The primary cause of tooth decay is poor mouth hygiene. Thus, tooth decay isn't inevitable; you can prevent it by following the guidelines covered in Chapter 1. Some causes of tooth decay are less easily avoided. Illnesses that cause repeated vomiting can lead to tooth decay. How? The stomach's contents are very acidic and can eat away a tooth's enamel, leaving it susceptible to decay. Several factors can determine the effects of prolonged vomiting, including the thickness of the tooth's enamel, the number of other acids attacking the tooth, and the frequency and duration of the vomiting. During such an illness, you should continue mouth hygiene.

How decay spreads

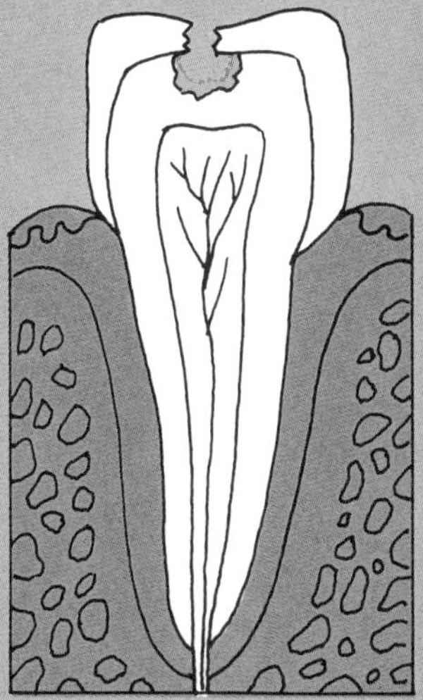

Acid starts decay...

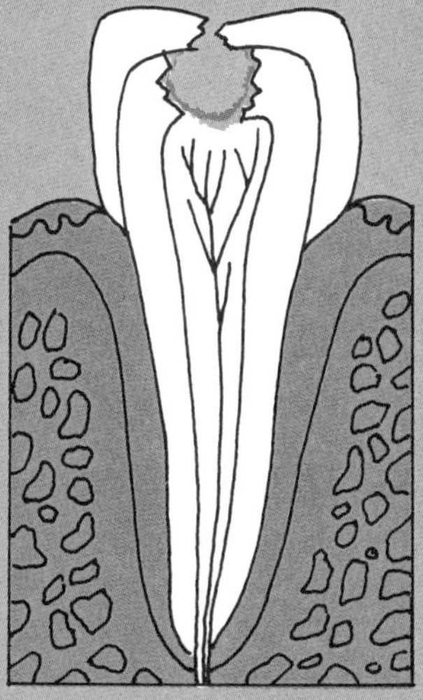

and eats into dentin...

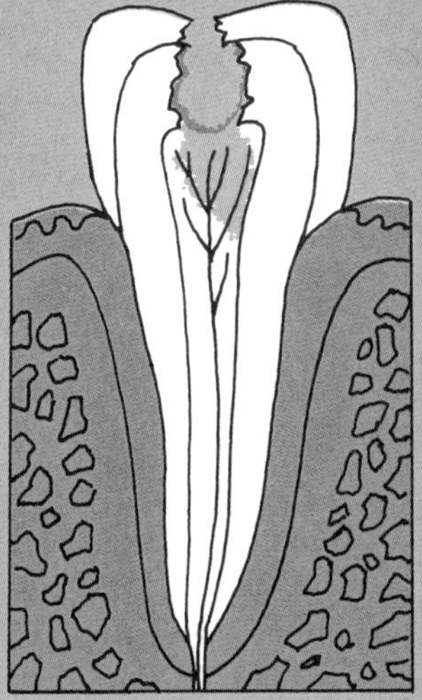

until the pulp becomes inflamed, causing pain.

See your dentist
If you visit your dentist regularly—twice a year is the recommended schedule—he'll detect your cavities in their early stages. You'll thus avoid extensive dental work.

Detecting cavities

During your regular checkup, your dentist will examine your teeth for early signs of decay. Most dentists use a mirror and a needle-shaped probe to look and feel for any color changes or cracks that might indicate the beginning of a cavity. Cavities can also be detected by X-rays.

When your dentist finds and repairs a cavity at an early stage, the decay is stopped and no further damage need occur. Having regular checkups keeps you certain that cavities don't go undetected. If you don't visit your dentist, the first sign of a cavity may be pain—an indication that the decay has spread.

How a cavity undermines a tooth

Once bacteria can pass through the hard enamel, they'll eat through the dentin. If the decay isn't treated, the bacteria will reach the pulp and destroy it.

If the pulp becomes infected with decay, pus may form. Infected pus at the base of the tooth can then form an abscess. The pus may spread into the jawbone and erode a small canal, or sinus, through the bone and gum. When the pus reaches the gum, it causes a swelling, called a boil.

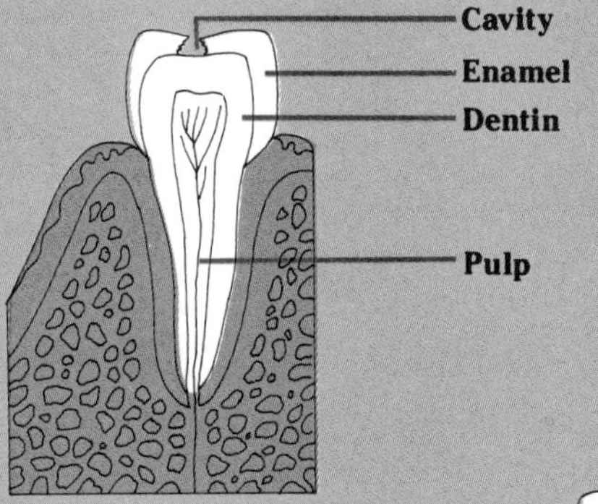

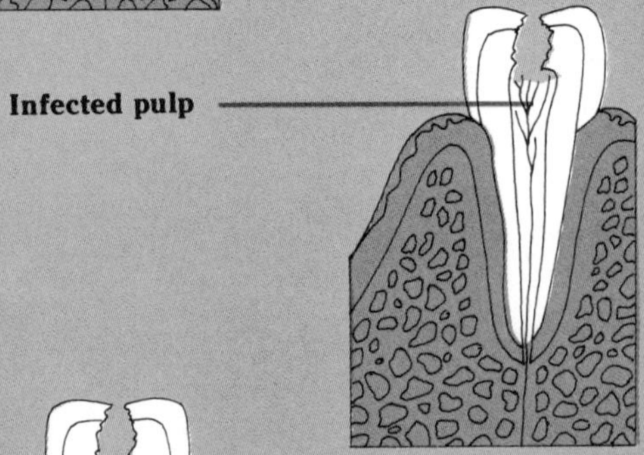

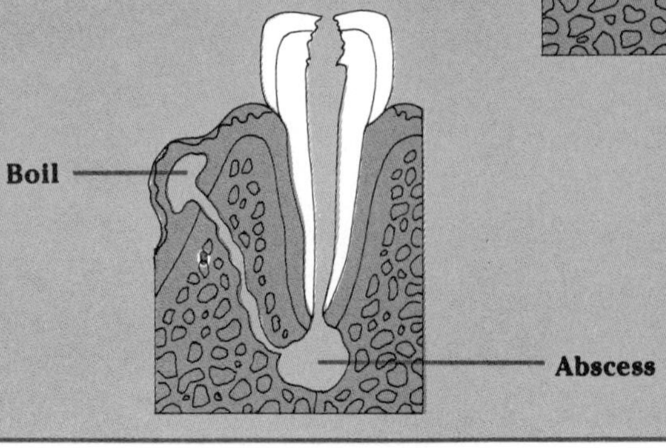

Types of cavities

Cavities can be divided into four general types, according to where they occur on the tooth. The four types are:

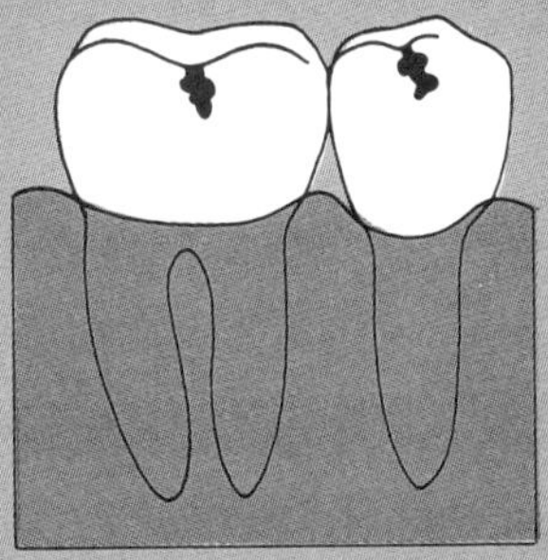

• ***Pit and fissure cavities***, the most common type. They occur in the pits and fissures—nooks and crevices—of teeth, the areas in and around teeth that are hard to reach during cleaning, where bacteria gather and multiply.

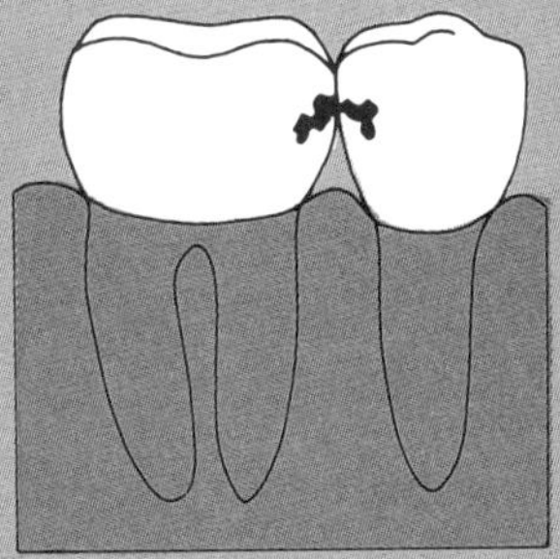

• ***Smooth-surface cavities***, between two teeth where food particles collect and cause damage if you don't floss. X-rays are usually necessary to spot a smooth-surface cavity.

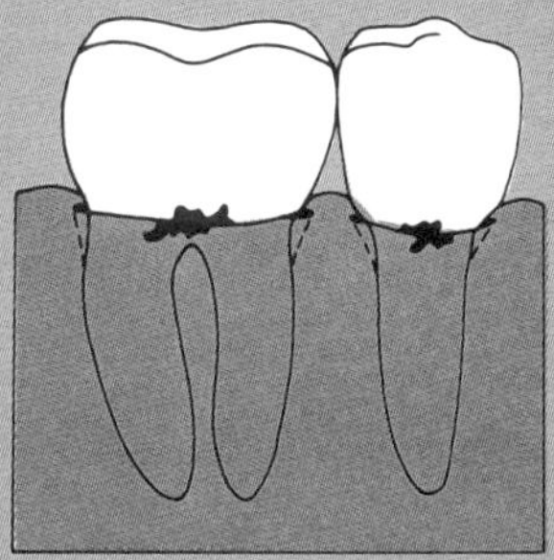

• ***Gumline cavities***, along a tooth beneath the gumline. As plaque builds up, the gum can become irritated and pull away from a tooth. Plaque then spreads into the exposed area, and a cavity can form beneath the gumline.

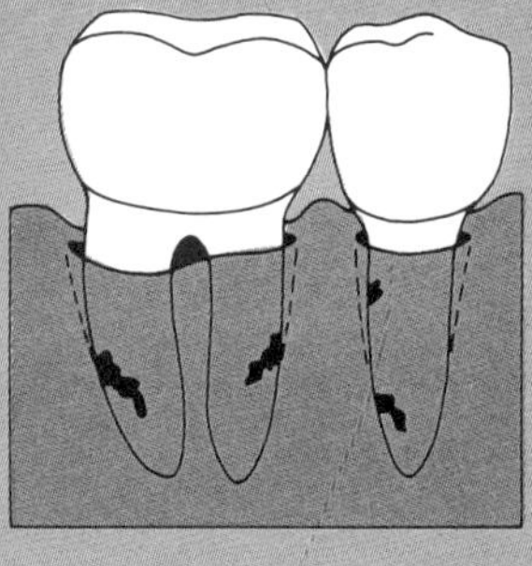

• ***Root cavities***, most often in older people who maintain poor oral hygiene. Because plaque isn't cleaned away, it builds up and irritates the gum. In time, the gum recedes to such an extent that the tooth's root is exposed and attacked by bacteria. A root cavity differs from a cavity that begins on the outside enamel and works its way through the tooth to the root.

A tooth's five surfaces

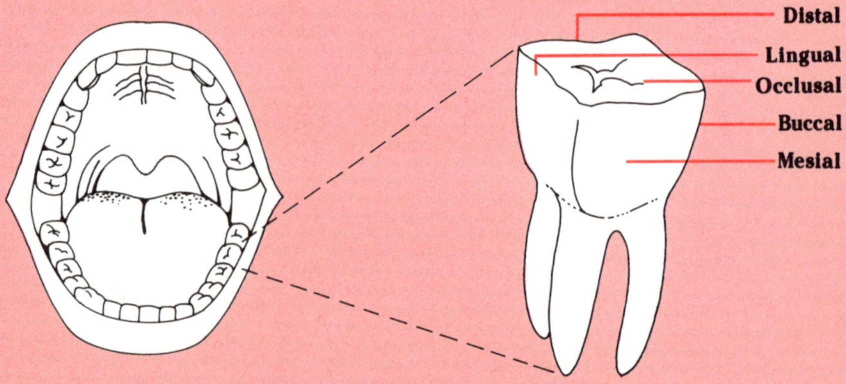

Proximal cavities
Cavities on mesial and distal surfaces are called proximal cavities.

Dentists further divide cavities into five classes. The purpose of these five classes is to determine exactly where on the tooth the cavity lies; each class is treated and repaired according to a slightly different procedure. These classes are based on the five surfaces of each tooth:

- occlusal: on the chewing surface
- lingual: on the surface that faces the tongue
- buccal: on the surface that faces the lips or cheek
- mesial: on the surface between two teeth that faces the front of the mouth
- distal: on the surface between two teeth that faces the back of the mouth.

Does a cavity always have to be filled?
Your dentist will fill a tooth if the enamel has been damaged. If the tooth's surface protection isn't restored, bacteria can enter the tooth and destroy the dentin and, if not stopped, can move on to destroy the pulp.

Repairing tooth decay

Your dentist will classify your cavity and determine the correct treatment according to which surface—or combination of surfaces—the cavity occurs on and which tooth—or teeth—is affected.

In repairing tooth decay, your dentist removes the tooth's decayed portion and restores the tooth to its natural shape and proper function. The treatment your dentist selects will depend on the extent of the decay.

If the cavity isn't too deep or the tooth isn't too severely decayed, your dentist will remove the decayed portion and replace it with a filling; if the tooth is severely decayed, he may use a premade filling that he'll cement into the tooth (an inlay); if the tooth has several cavities and can't be filled but the base of the tooth and its roots are healthy, he may install an artificial crown.

These measures involve drilling the tooth and removing the decayed portion, activities that would be very uncomfortable without an anesthetic.

Fundamentals of decay repair

The process of decay repair starts when the dentist locates a cavity and determines the extent of decay.

To repair the cavity, the dentist first drills the tooth's decayed part, taking care to remove all the decayed material.

He then fills the cavity and restores the tooth's original shape with an amalgam filling, inlay, onlay, or crown, as appropriate.

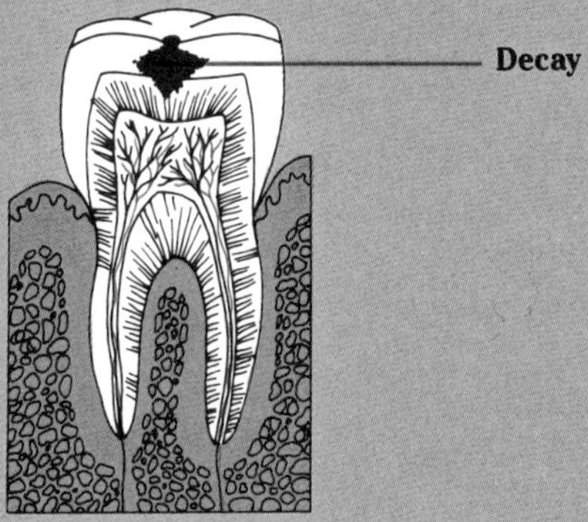

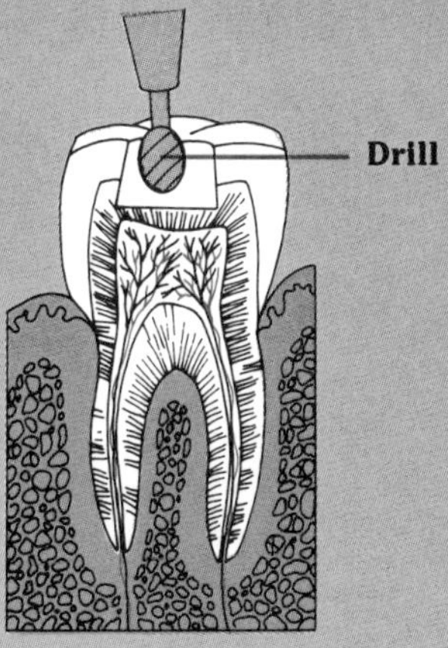

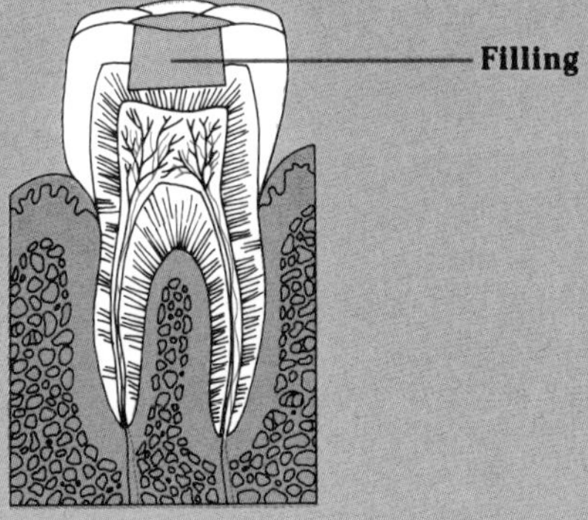

Benzocaine
Benzocaine in sprays and creams alleviates the pain and burning of minor cuts and burns.

Anesthetics

Before drilling out a cavity, your dentist will probably give you a local anesthetic to minimize your discomfort during treatment. He'll inject an anesthetic into your mouth in the area of the decayed tooth. Before giving you the injection, your dentist may apply a topical anesthetic to the skin's surface where he'll insert the needle. The topical anesthetic makes the

Major facial nerves and their anesthetic injection sites

Nerves	Lower jaw areas
Buccal	Buccal tissue of molars
Lingual	Back two thirds of tongue from molars to midline
Inferior alveolar (includes dental, mental, and incisive branches)	Molars, premolars, cuspids, incisors, and supporting structures; chin and lower lip
Mental branch of inferior alveolar	Chin and lower lip
Incisive and mental branches of inferior alveolar	Premolars, cuspids, incisors, and supporting structures; jaw and lower lip
Individual terminal branches of mental and incisive	Individual cuspids, incisors, and sometimes premolars; facial tissue and lip overlying individual teeth
Anterior portion of lingual nerve	Tongue in area of injection
Free nerve endings	Individual soft-tissue nerve endings
	Upper jaw areas
Greater palatine	Roof of mouth
Nasopalatine	Roof of mouth
Posterior superior alveolar	Second and third molars; first molar (partial); surrounding and overlying tissues
Middle superior alveolar (MSA) branch of the infraorbital nerve	First and second premolars; first molar (partial), supporting structures and overlying tissues; cheek and lip
Anterior superior alveolar (ASA) branch of the infraorbital nerve	Cuspids and incisors and supporting structures; overlying facial tissues and lip
Infraorbital (includes both MSA and ASA)	Premolars, cuspids, incisors, and supporting structures; overlying facial tissue, cheek, and lip
Individual branches of MSA or ASA	Individual premolars, cuspids, incisors, and supporting structures; facial tissue and lip overlying individual teeth
Free nerve endings	Individual soft-tissue nerve endings

Allergic reactions
In years past, novocaine was widely used by dentists, and allergic reactions were common. Today, lidocaine (Xylocaine) is used most often, and allergic reactions occur much less frequently.

local anesthetic injection less painful. The topical anesthetic is often a form of benzocaine or lidocaine in an ointment or cream form; the dentist applies it with a cotton swab.

After applying the topical anesthetic, your dentist will inject the local anesthetic. The area around the injection site will soon become numb, but before he begins to work your dentist will probably check to

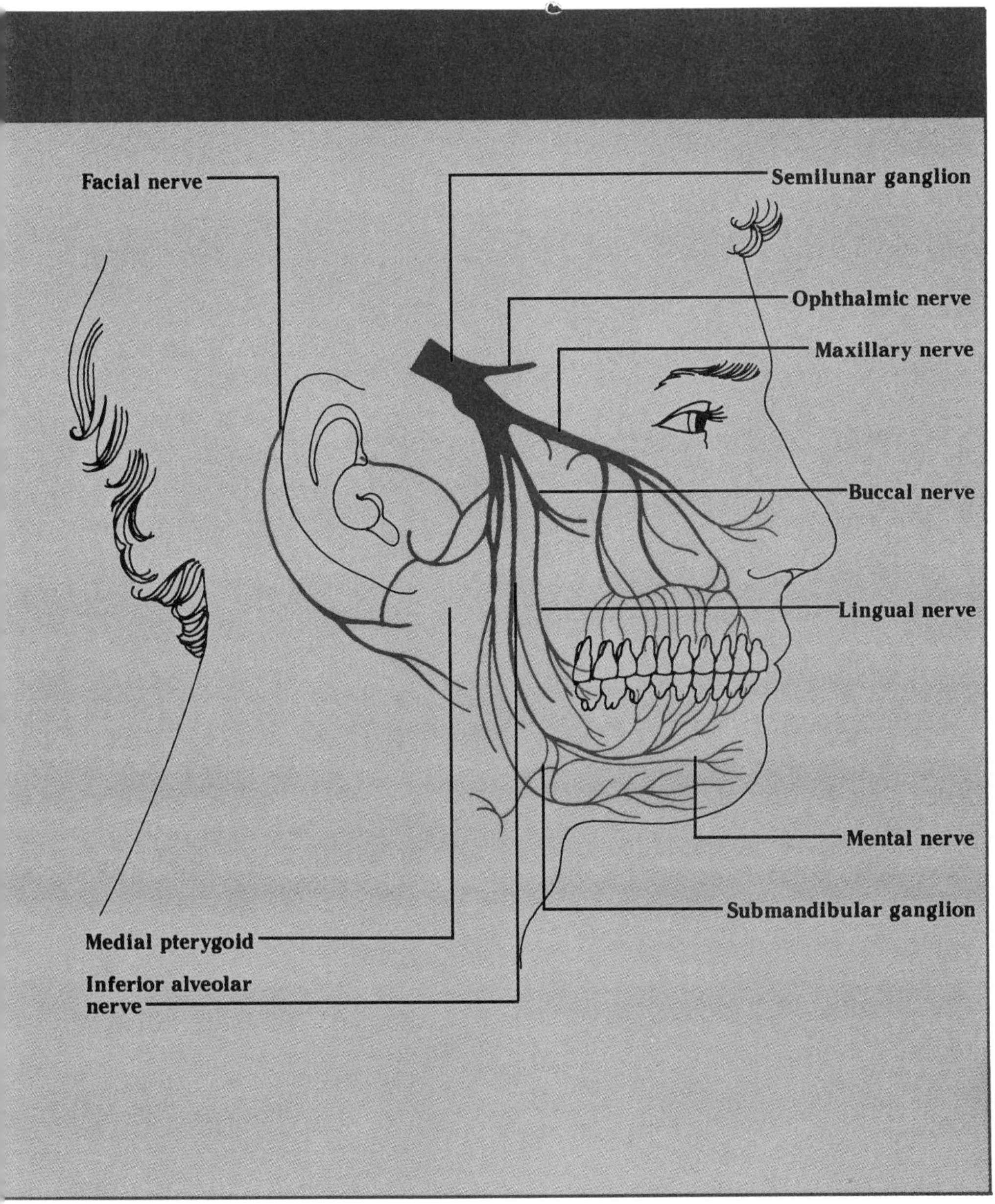

Local versus general anesthetics

A local anesthetic affects only the area directly surrounding the injection site; a general anesthetic affects your entire body. Because most general anesthetics put you to sleep, they're used mostly for more extensive procedures.

Common reactions to local anesthesia

Although short-lived negative reactions to local anesthetics sometimes occur, they usually aren't serious and don't require medical attention. Some of the most common temporary reactions include:

- *facial paralysis from a misdirected upper-lower jaw injection, producing such effects as inability to close the eyelid and drooping of the mouth*
- *blurred or double vision from entry of anesthetic into the optic nerve from an upper jaw injection*
- *bleeding from puncture of a blood vessel during injection; bleeding commonly follows a posterior superior alveolar injection done to anesthetize the lower jaw molars.*
- *localized tissue damage from injection of excessive amounts of anesthetic*
- *jaw pain and difficulty opening the mouth, commonly occurring after an inferior alveolar nerve injection*
- *prolonged numbness or tingling, possibly caused by nerve damage from a misdirected needle or, rarely, by a contaminated anesthetic solution.*

see if you still have any feeling there. If you do, your dentist may give you additional medication. Some people respond less to the effects of anesthetics than others.

Some people experience allergic reactions to certain anesthetics, and some people, particularly those with heart conditions, high blood pressure, thyroid conditions, or diabetes, may experience other adverse reactions to certain anesthetics. Both novocaine and the more widely used lidocaine (Xylocaine) must be used with a vasoconstrictor, such as epinephrine (Adrenalin). A vasoconstrictor is a compound that makes blood vessels smaller (constricted). By making blood vessels smaller, the vasoconstrictor helps the anesthetic remain where it's injected: the anesthetic is less likely to travel from the injection site through the constricted vessels and lasts longer. Unfortunately, vasoconstrictors can cause problems for heart patients, blood pressure patients, and people with thyroid conditions or diabetes. An alternative exists for such people: mepivacaine, an anesthetic that works without a vasoconstrictor.

Another aid many dentists use to make your time in the chair less difficult is nitrous oxide, more commonly known as laughing gas. Nitrous oxide can be especially helpful for you if going to the dentist makes you nervous or upset. While it doesn't eliminate pain the way an anesthetic does, nitrous oxide can put you in such a relaxed state that the sensations you feel simply won't bother you. Nitrous oxide is administered through a small mask that fits over your nose. The mixture is at least 20% oxygen to 80% nitrous oxide. As the amount of oxygen is increased, the effects of the nitrous oxide decrease. If you want to try this alternative, talk it over with your dentist.

4 Having Fillings, Inlays, and Crowns

Chemical drilling

Is painless drilling possible? Impossible? Well, some dentists now offer an alternative to the high-speed drill—an instrument known as the chemical drill. Instead of removing the tooth's decayed part with a drill bit, your dentist would use a chemical drill that gently washes away decay with a warm liquid. An anesthetic isn't needed because the procedure is painless. (Some conventional high-speed drilling may be necessary, however, to reach all the decay or to complete the preparation for the filling material.)

Once the anesthetic or nitrous oxide has taken effect, your dentist will begin working with a high-speed, water-cooled drill. Your dentist uses the drill to make a hole through the tooth's enamel surface to the decayed dentin. Having exposed the decayed area, he'll remove all decay traces and then flush the hole with water and air. Then he'll probably use a different drill to shape the hole so that the filling will stay in place. By shaping the hole correctly, the dentist makes sure the filling will remain in the hole even under the stress of everyday chewing.

Fillings

The kind of material used to restore a tooth—to fill the hole created by drilling and removing decay—will depend on the tooth's location. The filling used in an easily visible tooth usually differs from that used in a less visible tooth. Cost, too, may be a factor. An expensive gold filling in a baby tooth would be a waste of money since the child will lose the tooth in a short time.

The old and the new

Dentistry has come a long way since Dr. G.V. Black patented the first dental drill (shown at left) in 1871. This foot-powered contraption was known as a "tooth-dressing machine."

In contrast, a new drill (shown at right) features a fiberoptic light that eliminates shadows, flowing water to cool the drill bit, and variable drilling speeds.

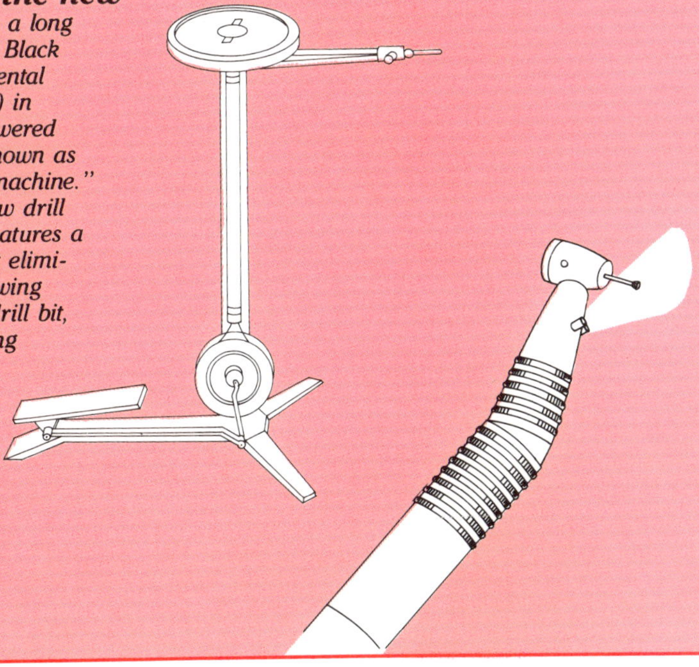

Gold

Gold is used for large cavities because it resists corrosion and is stronger and less sensitive to temperature changes than amalgam. On the negative side, gold is expensive, and many people don't find gold teeth attractive.

The material used for most fillings is silver amalgam—a mixture of several metals, usually mercury, silver, tin, copper, and zinc. Silver amalgam is best in a tooth with enough solid tooth structure to hold and support the filling material. For deep holes, a cement or varnish base may be necessary as insulation before the filling material goes in place. A still larger hole will require different material and procedures.

Your dentist will use special tools to put the silver amalgam in place and pack it into the hole. A few minutes after it's inserted, the material will begin to harden. At this point, your dentist will carve the filling material to match the shape of your tooth. To make certain the filling is correctly formed, he'll place a small piece of articulating paper (it looks like carbon paper) on your new filling and ask you to bite down. Any colored marks left on the new filling indicate that more carving is needed.

Silver amalgam is commonly used on back teeth. If the hole to be filled is on a front tooth, you'll probably want a filling material that matches the tooth's color. The preferred material for filling front teeth is a composite of barium, lithium, quartz or silica, and acrylic. This material looks like tooth enamel but, unfortunately, it wears down faster than amalgam fillings and may stain more easily than your natural enamel.

Mountains in your mouth

The contact between your upper and lower teeth is extremely sensitive. If a filling is only 5 mm (approximately 0.2 inch) too high, it can feel mountainous. In fact, it can cause problems later by changing your bite. (The importance of a well-aligned bite is discussed further on pages 58, 74, and 75.)

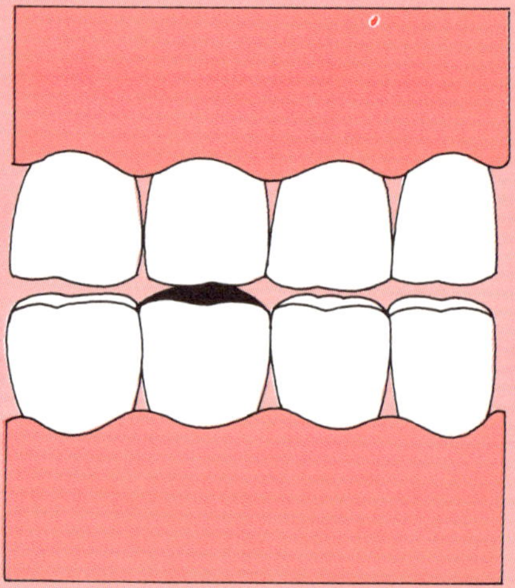

How a dentist fills a cavity

A cavity is a hole through a tooth's enamel. If the cavity isn't filled, the decay may spread to the dentin and from there attack the tooth's pulp. Your dentist will drill a hole into the tooth, remove all traces of decay, and then shape the hole so that it will securely hold the filling.

If the tooth's in the back of your mouth, your dentist will fill the hole with silver amalgam; if the tooth's in the front of your mouth or is easily visible, he'll fill it with a tooth-colored material.

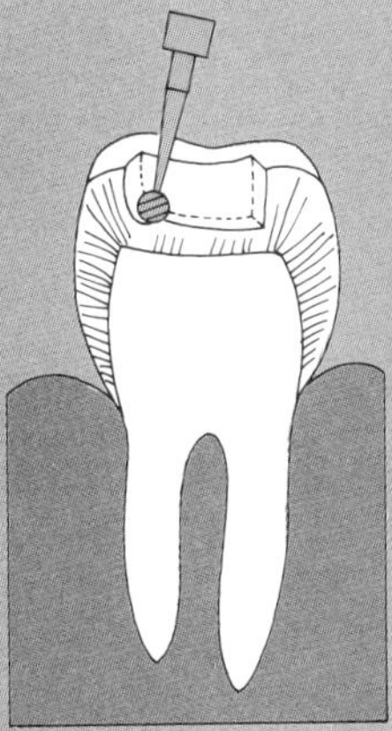

Drilling into decay

Once the dentist has completely prepared the cavity, he mixes the silver amalgam—equal portions of metal filings and mercury. He then packs the amalgam into the cavity with a special tool. When he's completely filled the cavity, the dentist carves the amalgam to the proper contour.

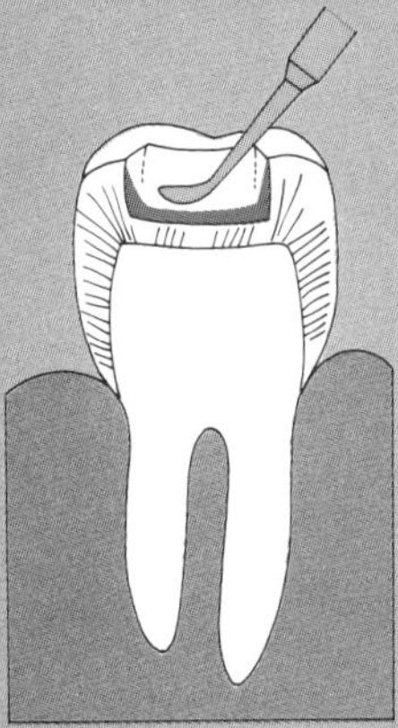

Packing the filling

Then he polishes it to ensure a smooth, tight fit.

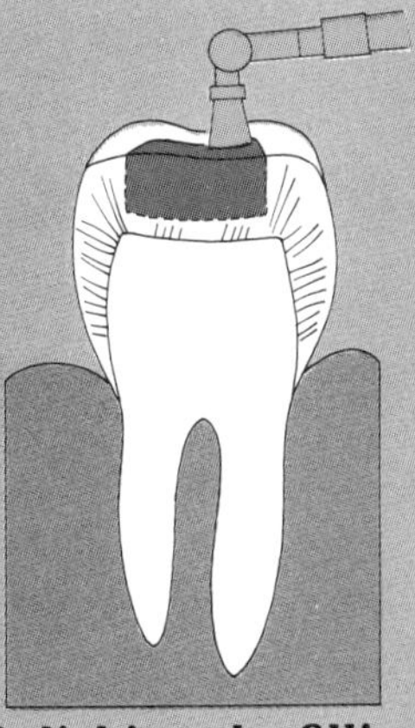

Polishing the filling

Inlay–onlay: What's the difference?
An inlay's a filling made outside your mouth after your dentist drills the decayed tooth and makes an impression of the hole to be filled. If the decay's so widespread that the tooth's walls may not support an inlay, then an onlay may be the answer. An onlay's a filling made outside your mouth, too, but it extends over the edges of the repaired tooth, protecting the tooth's walls.

Inlays

If the cavity is large, removal of the decay may not leave enough tooth structure to support a standard filling: an inlay—a filling made outside your tooth—may be necessary. Most inlays are made of gold. After your dentist removes the decay, he'll make a wax impression of the cavity and order a prepared filling from a dental laboratory. He'll cement this prepared filling into the cavity. You'll have a temporary filling while the inlay is being made.

When the gold inlay is ready, your dentist will remove the temporary filling and put the gold inlay in place to test the fit. He'll make the necessary adjustments for the inlay to fit the space perfectly. When the fitting is completed, your dentist will cement the inlay in place, test your bite with articulating paper, and polish the surface.

To prepare a gold inlay, a dental laboratory technician makes a plaster cast of the wax impression your dentist has taken. He then pours hot wax into the cast to make a wax pattern of the cavity. Next,

Preparing an inlay
After he's drilled the tooth, your dentist takes an impression of the tooth and the drilled hole. He sends the impression to a laboratory that makes the inlay. Your dentist perfects the inlay's fit in your tooth. Then he cements it permanently in place and polishes the surface.

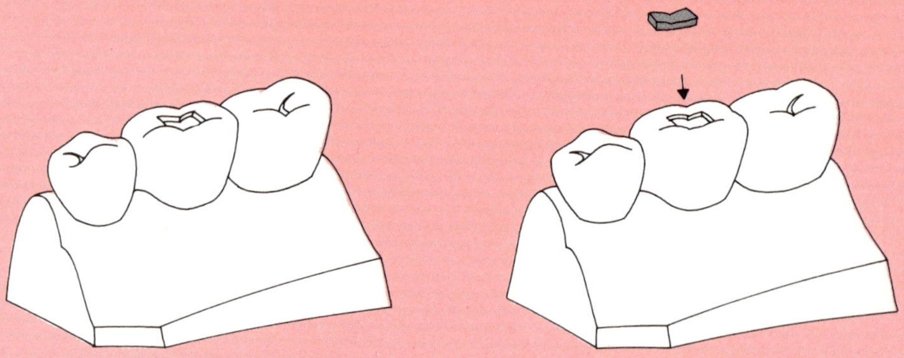

he makes a gold casting of the wax pattern; when the molten gold has cooled, he polishes it to a high gloss and sends it to your dentist for fitting.

Onlays

If a cavity is too large even for an inlay, your dentist may decide that you need an onlay. Like an inlay, an onlay is made outside your mouth from a wax pattern and, when cemented in place, actually strengthens your tooth by supporting the remaining tooth structure. The difference between an onlay and an inlay is that the onlay extends over the cusp edges of the tooth's biting surface, whereas an inlay is confined within the heights of the cusps. An inlay is used when the decayed area is small; an onlay, when decay is extensive or if the tooth has previously been filled.

An onlay is often used in place of a full crown; some dentists feel that since an onlay contacts less gum area than a full crown, it makes the gum less susceptible to gingivitis and the tooth less susceptible to recurrent decay.

Preparing an onlay

After he's drilled the tooth, your dentist takes an impression of the tooth. He sends the impression to a laboratory that makes the onlay. Your dentist perfects the onlay's fit on your tooth. Then he cements it in place.

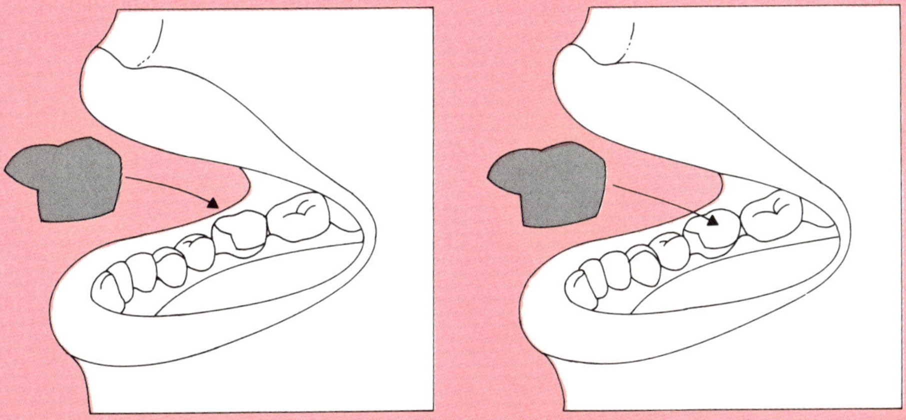

Crowns

If a tooth has several cavities or is severely decayed, a filling or an inlay may not be usable. Your dentist may recommend an artificial crown, sometimes called a cap. (A crown can also cover a broken [fractured] tooth or a chipped tooth.) Most crowns are made of gold or some other metal that is covered partly or entirely with porcelain.

Porcelain caps wear down slowly but are breakable. Porcelain over gold or some other metal offers the strength of the metal and the appearance of the porcelain. Gold alone is durable and won't break like porcelain, but many people don't want a visible gold cap. Discuss the advantages, disadvantages, and cost of each with your dentist.

A crown is a hollow shell fitted over the old tooth and cemented in place. A mold (impression) is made of the tooth to determine the shape of the crown; your dentist may also file the tooth down to make the crown fit more easily. You'll wear a temporary plastic crown until your permanent crown is ready.

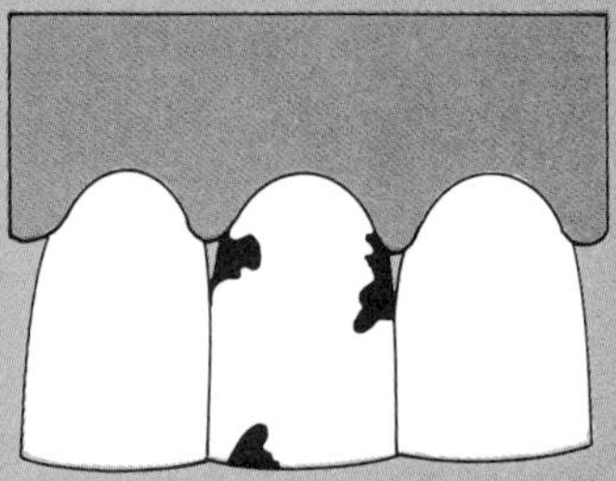

If a tooth has too many cavities...

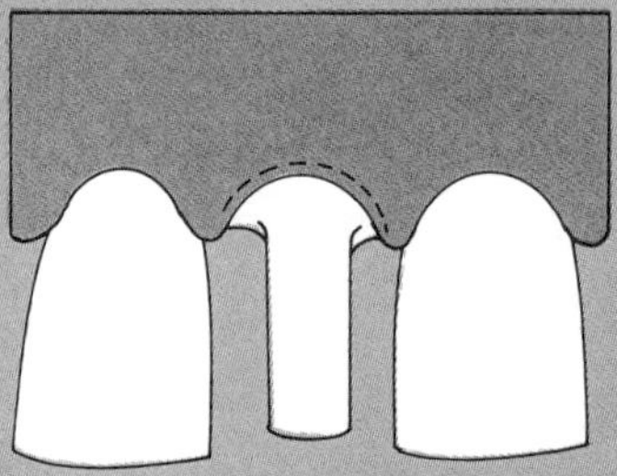

your dentist may drill the tooth down to a post, take an impression...

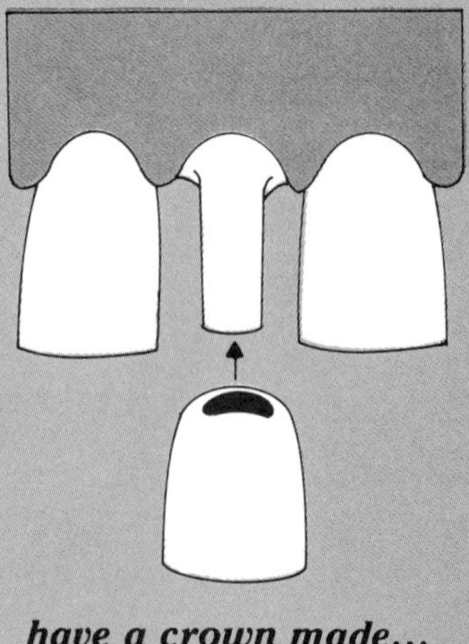

have a crown made...

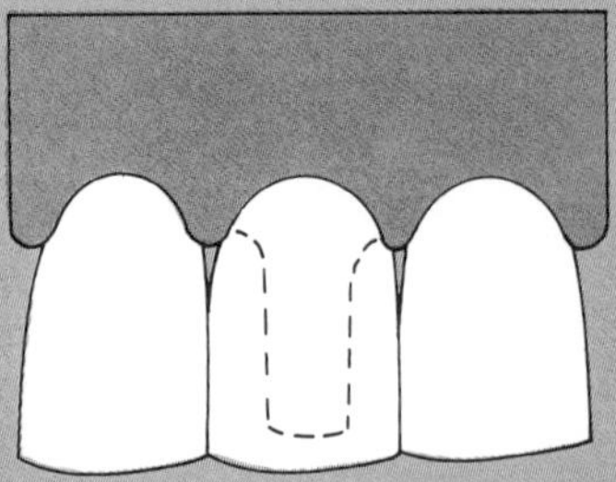

and fit the crown over the tooth post.

Post crowns

A tooth may be so badly decayed or weakened that it isn't strong enough to hold a crown. In this case, your dentist may insert a metal post into the tooth to hold the crown.

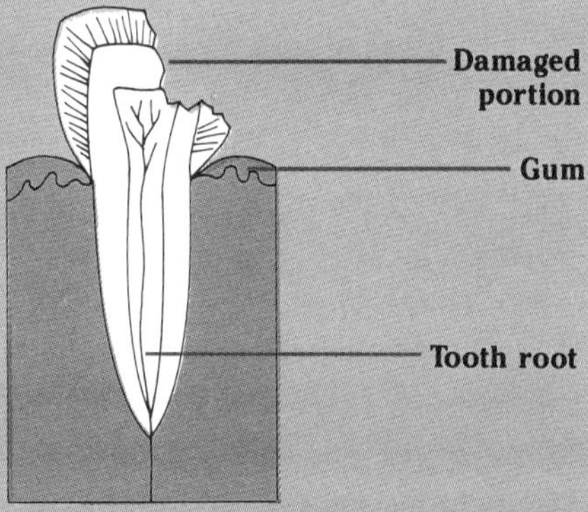

First, the dentist trims the tooth down to the gumline. This involves removal of any remaining portions of the crown. Next, he'll remove the tooth's pulp from the root's canal and treat the canal with an antiseptic. Then, he'll shape the canal and take an impression of it. This impression is used to create an ice-cream-cone–shaped post (most posts are made of gold).

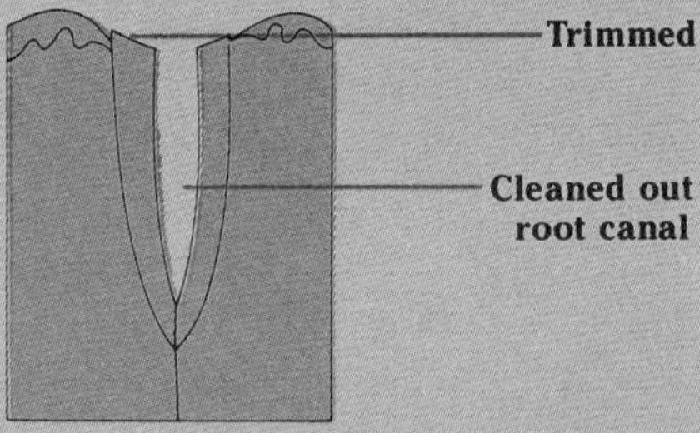

Finally, he'll fit the post securely into the root canal, fit the post with a crown, and attach the crown to the post.

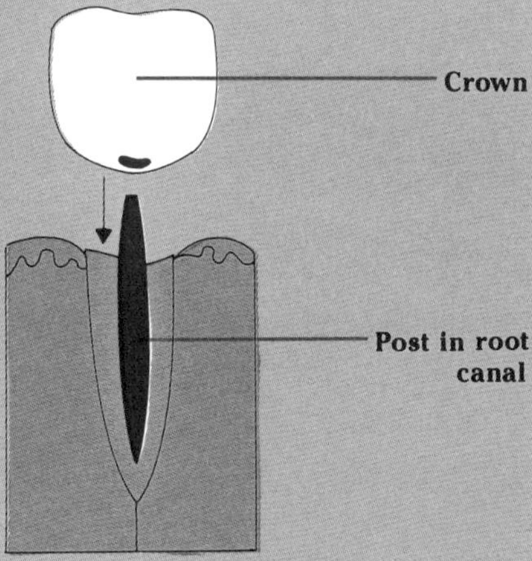

Today, many dentists use stainless-steel posts instead of gold posts. Because these posts don't need to be cast to match the shape of the root canal, they save time and expense.

5 Correcting Gum Diseases

Properly cared for, your teeth will last your lifetime. Indeed, the most common cause of tooth loss, disease of the surrounding tissues (periodontal disease), is preventable.

What's around a tooth

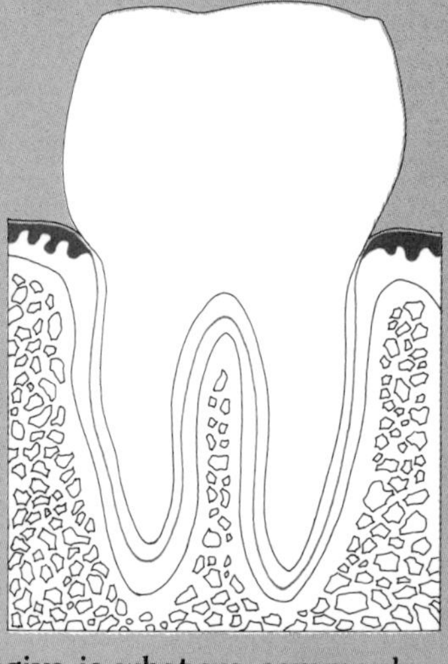

Gingiva is what we commonly refer to as gums. Gums surround the neck of each tooth, providing support, insulation, and some protection from bacteria.

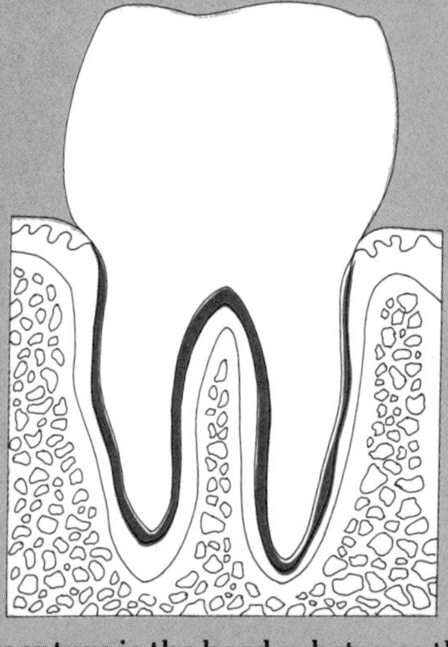

Cementum is the hard substance that surrounds and protects the root of each tooth.

Periodontal tissue

Periodontal means "around the tooth" and refers to the structures that support teeth. The root of each tooth is supported by periodontal tissue, or periodontium. This tissue actually consists of four separate tissues: gingiva, cementum, alveolar process, and periodontal ligament.

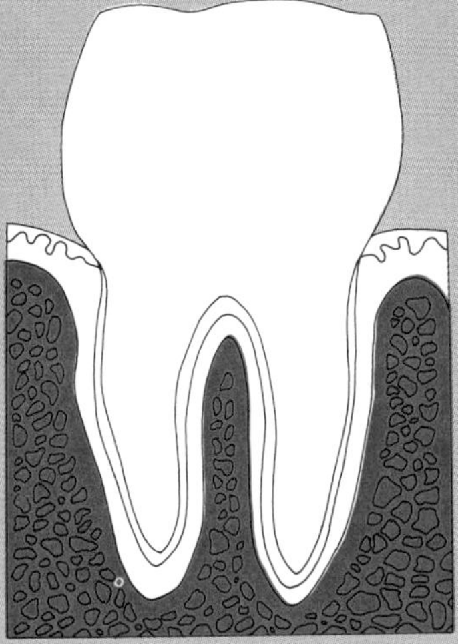

The alveolar process is the bone that forms the sockets teeth rest in. This alveolar bone is constantly dissolved and replaced by new bone, a process caused by the pressure exerted on the teeth because of their positioning. This constant reforming of the alveolar bone explains why teeth can be made to assume new positions, as when they're realigned—the alveolar bone reforms itself to hold the teeth in the new position.

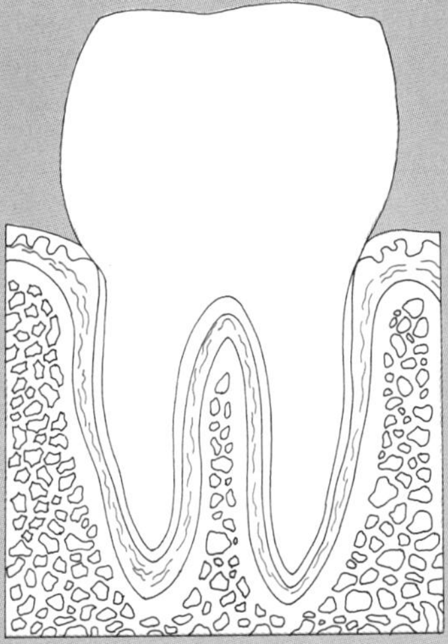

The periodontal ligament connects each tooth's root to its socket and protects the dentin. The periodontal ligament is located outside the cementum.

Tooth loss
The major cause of tooth loss for most adults over age 40 is severe inflammation of the gums caused by the buildup of plaque and tartar—periodontal disease. Unfortunately, 95% of children aged 5 to 15 already have some degree of gum trouble.

Periodontal disease

Periodontal, or gum, disease destroys the tissues that support teeth; left untreated, periodontal disease can result in the loss of even cavity-free teeth. Over half of all adults over age 18 experience at least the early stages of periodontal disease, but the disease isn't restricted to adults. In recent years, dentists have reported an increasing number of teenagers and young children with gum problems.

Gingivitis

Gingivitis—inflamed and swollen gums—is the first stage of periodontal disease. This inflammation is

A close-up of gum disease

Both brushing and flossing help to remove plaque. Allowed to build up, plaque can lead to gum disease—and eventual tooth loss.

Healthy gums are pink and firm and fit tightly around the tooth.

Plaque buildup produces tartar that irritates the gums, which pull away from the tooth, causing a gum pocket—a place for more plaque buildup.

Bacteria spread down the tooth to the supporting bone.

The bacteria eat into the bone and tissue that surround and anchor the tooth. The gum becomes more irritated and pulls further away from the tooth. These processes can loosen the tooth, which may eventually require extraction.

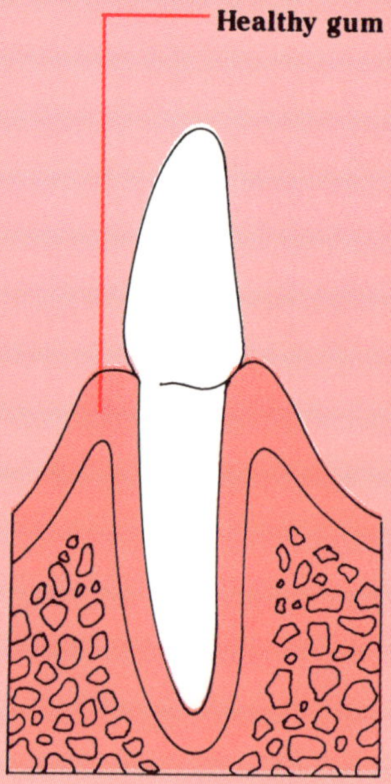

Children and gingivitis

Gingivitis is more common in adults and teenagers than in children, but children aren't immune to the disease. Young children who don't clean their teeth properly are susceptible to it.

caused by bacteria in plaque. Gingivitis affects only the soft, outer gum tissue and is reversible: most cases of gingivitis can be successfully treated by a dentist, and the gums will return to normal. However, because the disease isn't painful and develops slowly, a person may leave it untreated.

Left untreated, the disease spreads. As the gums become swollen, a space forms between the gum and the tooth. Bacteria invade this space, forming a diseased periodontal pocket. If this condition isn't treated by a dentist, the disease spreads further, developing into periodontitis.

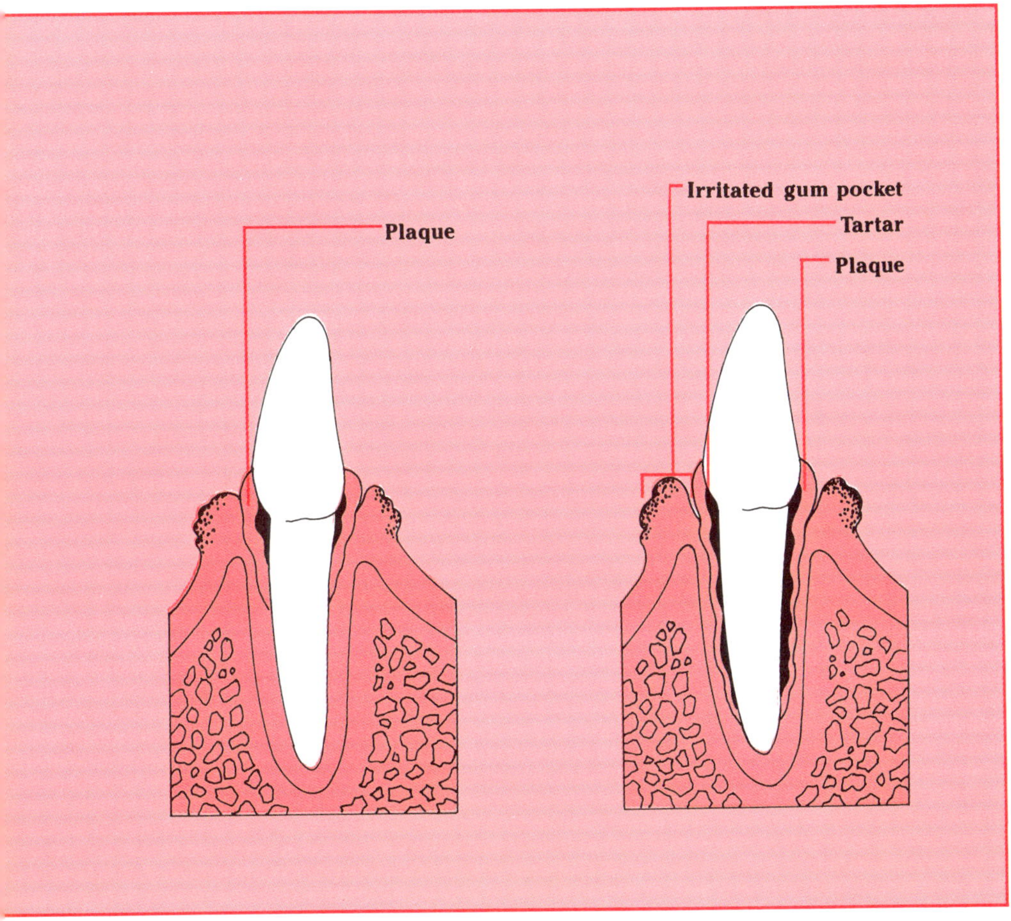

The stages of periodontal disease

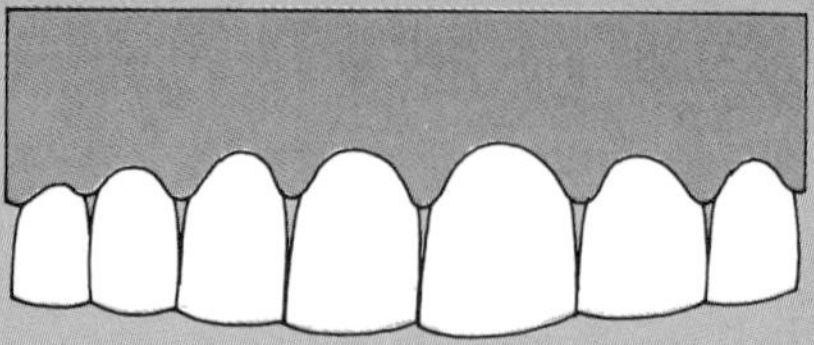

Normal gums can be undermined by plaque and tartar.

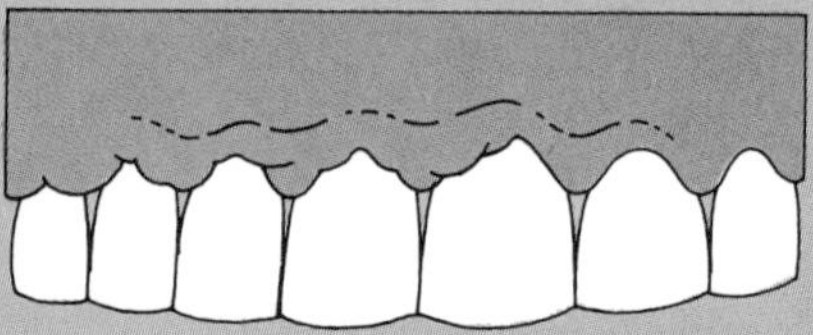

Inflamed gums become puffy and easily infected.

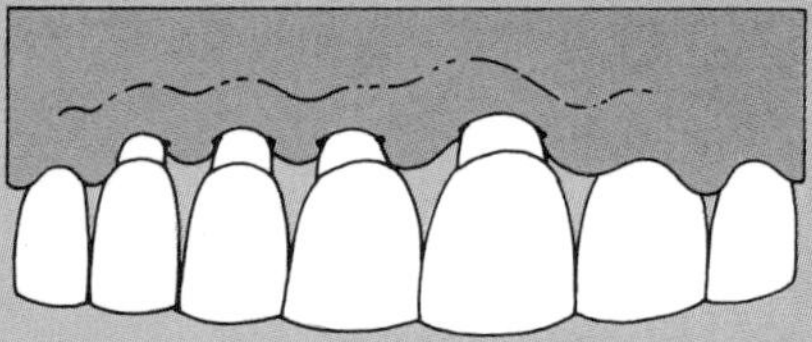

Irritated gums retreat, leaving spaces.

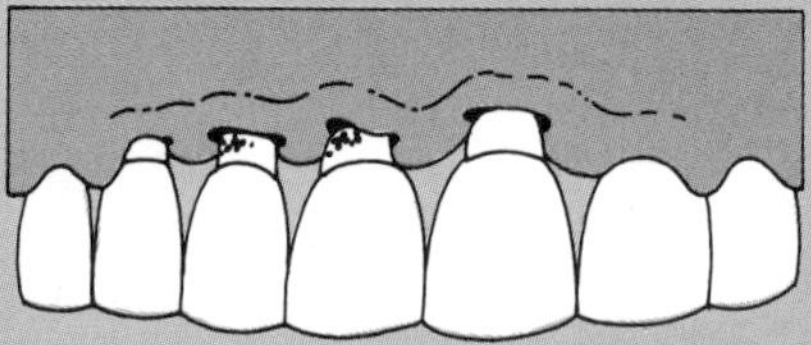

Bacteria invade, forming periodontal pockets.

Periodontitis

Periodontitis is the result of untreated gingivitis: the disease spreads from the gums to the bone that surrounds and supports the teeth. The teeth loosen in their sockets and begin to drift apart. Once the disease has reached this point, a specialist's intervention may be required.

Trench mouth

Trench mouth—also called acute gingivitis or Vincent's disease—is a painful infection and ulceration of the gums, usually between the teeth. Its name derives from World War I soldiers who fought in trenches. The conditions of trench warfare—constant stress, poor diet, and few opportunities to maintain good oral hygiene—promoted the growth of the bacteria that cause the infection.

Today, trench mouth is rare and usually afflicts teenagers and young adults. Too much stress, too much alcohol, excessive smoking, lack of sleep, and poor diet can weaken the body, opening the way to the growth of the bacteria that cause the disease. Trench mouth isn't believed to be contagious and is rarely dangerous, but it can occur quite suddenly and be painful.

The symptoms of trench mouth include swollen, bleeding gums; the gums take on a grayish color and become so tender that eating causes pain. As the disease progresses, ulcers form on the gums and bleed. You may also experience headaches or fever and have a metallic taste in your mouth along with bad breath. Brushing is painful because it removes the outer layer of the infection (the grayish color). However, the gray color will return quickly unless the disease is treated. A visit to your dentist is essential.

Treatment of trench mouth usually involves the use of an antibiotic to clear up the infection and a hydrogen peroxide rinse to relieve the pain and inflammation of the gums. Your dentist will scale the outer surface of your gums; after a few days, he'll scale under your gums. This scaling process may have to be repeated. Your dentist will then prescribe a rigorous routine of oral hygiene and will probably suggest that you make some changes in your life-style, such as eating properly and getting enough rest.

Trench mouth
Trench mouth is an acute form of gum inflammation (gingivitis). As trench mouth develops, ulcers form in the mouth, particularly on the already inflamed gums.

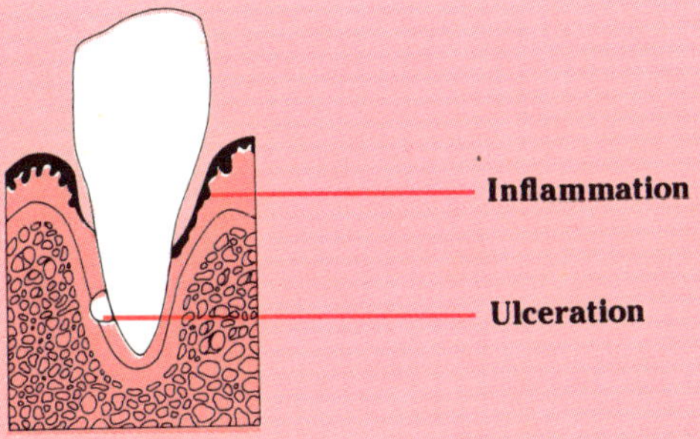

Calculus: Tartar by another name

Calculus, or tartar, results from the buildup of plaque. As plaque builds up, bacteria in the deeper layers die and mineralize, forming calculus. You can prevent the growth of calculus by carefully brushing and flossing your teeth; but once a calculus forms, you'll need your dentist or dental hygienist to remove it. Some people develop deposits of calculus no matter how carefully they clean their teeth—such people must visit their dentist every few months to have the calculus removed.

Causes of periodontal disease

By far the most common cause of gum disease is the buildup of plaque, the bacteria-containing film that forms on teeth.

Plaque contains irritants that damage gums and cause them to become inflamed and swollen—gingivitis. If not removed, plaque builds up and forms a hard deposit, called calculus or tartar. As more plaque forms on top of the calculus, the gums pull away from the teeth, forming small spaces. Bacteria then move into these spaces, causing an infection. As the disease progresses, it spreads along the roots of the teeth to the supporting bones—resulting in periodontitis.

Several other factors can increase the risk or severity of periodontal disease. People who smoke or chew tobacco are more likely to develop periodontal disease—and develop more severe cases of it—than are people who don't use tobacco.

Smoking can decrease the blood flow to your gums, making them less healthy. Furthermore, nicotine encourages plaque buildup. Chewing tobacco is one of the most common causes of gum recession, part of the progression of periodontal disease. Chewing tobacco can also wear down the surfaces of teeth, the result of the "grit" in chewing tobacco.

Excessive drinking or ingestion of alcohol may dry out and burn the membranes of your mouth, killing cells. Alcohol abuse can also cause an imbalance of microorganisms in your mouth that will allow the growth of harmful bacteria.

Certain medications can have an adverse effect on your gums. These include oral contraceptives, some types of antiseizure drugs (such as Dilantin), steroids, and some cancer therapy drugs. Tell your dentist about any medications you're taking.

Any dental condition or bad oral habit that places abnormal stress or pressure on your teeth (trauma) can make your gums and supporting bone tissue more susceptible to periodontal disease.

Three causes of gum disease

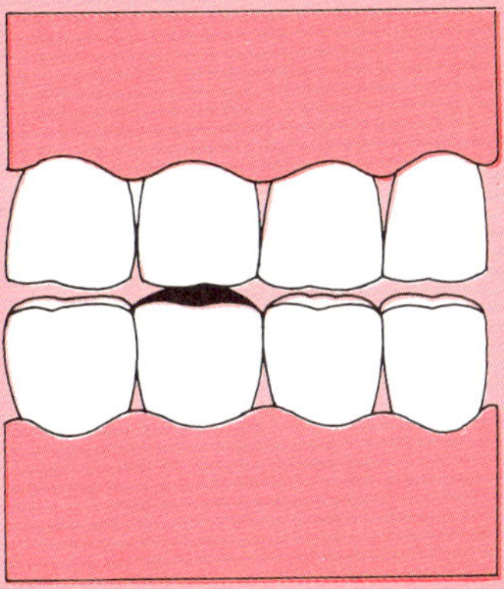

High or uneven filling

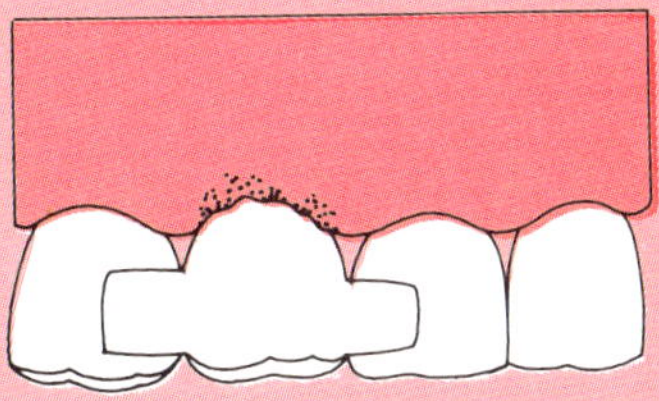

Bridge that doesn't fit properly

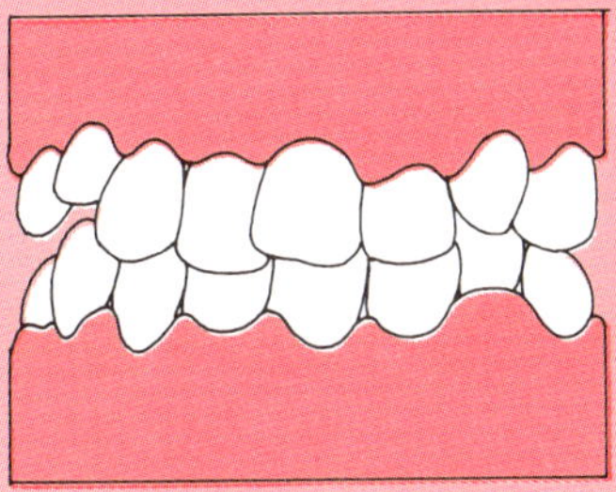

Poorly aligned teeth

Dental conditions (trauma) that can lead to gum disease include:

- malocclusions, also called occlusal traumatism (poorly aligned teeth)
- bridges or dentures that don't fit properly
- fillings that haven't been properly form-fitted and have too high or uneven surfaces.

Bad oral habits that can lead to gum disease include:

- nail or lip biting
- clenching or grinding your teeth (bruxism)
- use of toothpicks.

Heredity may also be a contributing factor to periodontal disease. If your parents are affected by it, the chances are increased that you, too, will be a candidate for the development of periodontal disease. You can't change your heredity, but you can be aware of your increased risk and take the proper preventive measures.

Pregnant women sometimes experience redness, tenderness, and swelling of their gums, results of changing hormone levels. The increase in hormones during pregnancy can exaggerate the reaction gums have to plaque. Pregnant women should visit the dentist regularly to have their teeth and gums checked.

Gauging periodontal damage

Your dentist will insert a periodontal probe into the space between the tooth and gum lining to assess the extent of gum detachment or bone loss. He'll measure each tooth this way.

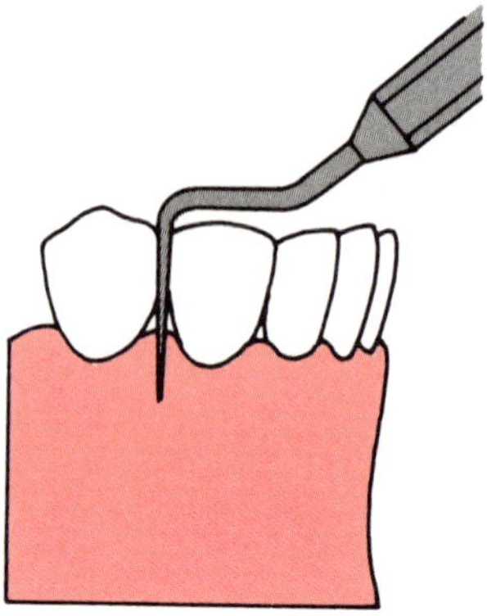

Dental problems and gum disease

Various dental problems can lead to periodontal disease. In malocclusion, poorly aligned teeth put extra pressure on and eventually weaken the periodontal ligament and the underlying bone. These weakened areas then become susceptible to the bacterial infection of periodontitis. Ill-fitting dentures can have the same effect. And overhanging rough margins on fillings and crowns irritate the gums and can provide a haven for infection-causing bacteria.

Symptoms of periodontal disease

Regular dental visits are essential to the prevention of periodontal disease. Periodontal disease usually progresses gradually for years without causing any major discomfort. Left untreated, it can cause permanent damage. If you wait until pain has started, the chances are that irreversible damage has been done.

Learn these warning signs of periodontal disease. See your dentist immediately if:

- your gums bleed regularly when you brush your teeth. Bleeding gums are an early symptom of gingivitis.
- your gums are red, swollen, or tender. Healthy gums are pale pink and firm; in gingivitis, they become red, soft, and swollen.
- your gums have pulled away from your teeth.
- pus comes out when you press gently on the margin of your gums.
- any permanent teeth are loose or separating.
- you notice any change in the way your teeth are aligned.
- you notice any changes in the way your partial dentures fit.
- you have chronic bad breath or an unpleasant taste in your mouth.

Treatment of periodontal disease

During your regular checkups, your dentist will examine your gums for any signs of periodontal problems. In the absence of irritated, swollen, or bleeding gums, the disease may be discovered by routine X-rays showing loss of bone surrounding the teeth. Your dentist may use a periodontal probe to check for any periodontal pockets that might have formed between your teeth and gums. He can also measure the depth of such pockets and judge the extent of damage.

Detected at an early stage, periodontal disease can be treated by your regular dentist. The treatment usually involves scaling the teeth to remove the plaque and calculus from the tooth surfaces, planing (smoothing) the root surfaces, and curettage—scraping plaque and inflamed tissue from the pockets that have formed around your teeth.

If the periodontal disease is advanced, you'll need to see a periodontist, a specialist in the diagnosis and treatment of gum disease.

Scaling, planing, and curettage

In scaling, the dentist uses a sickle-shaped hand scaler to scrape tartar from the tooth surface, particularly under the gum or near the gum margin.

Root planing involves smoothing the root of the tooth with a sharp curette. The dentist tries to get the root surface as smooth as possible to reduce plaque accumulation.

The dentist may also use the curette to remove plaque, calculus, and inflamed tissue from the gum pockets around each tooth—a process known as *curettage.*

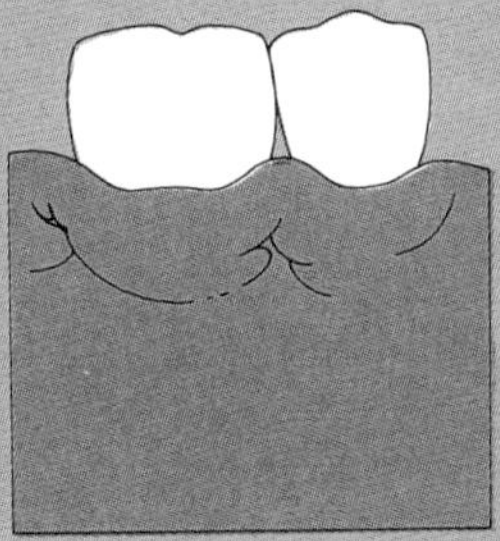

Inflamed gums

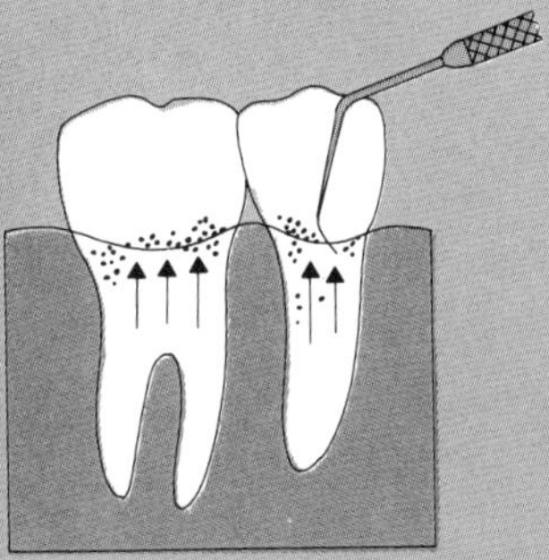

Root planing—using a curette from the tooth's root upward

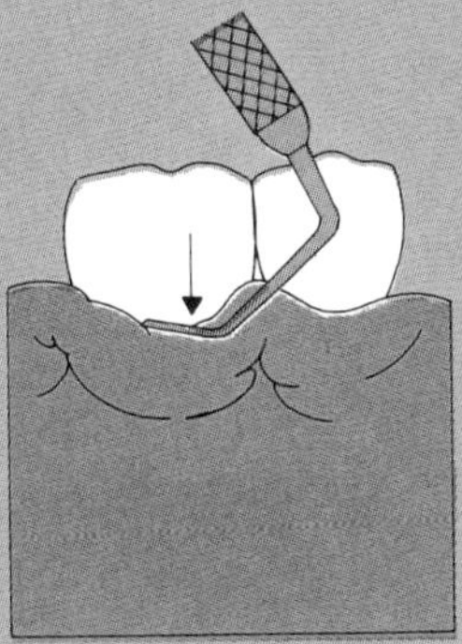

Scaling the tooth's surface

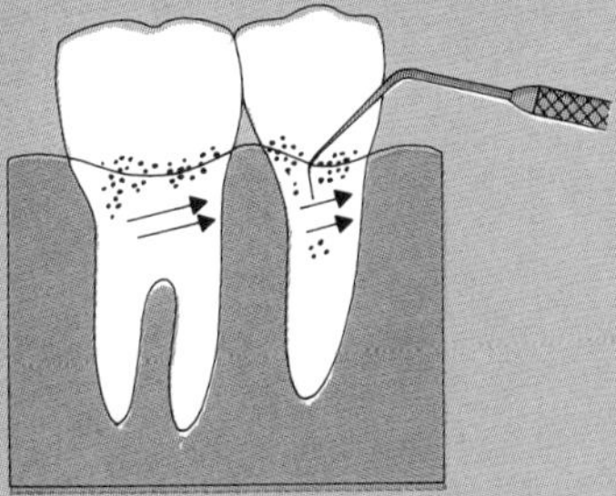

Using a curette across the root

Realignment of teeth

Because crooked, crowded, or protruding teeth can contribute to the development of periodontal disease, part of the treatment may involve therapy to realign your teeth.

Teeth that don't meet properly, an overbite, incorrectly fitted partial dentures, or a lost tooth that isn't replaced can cause damage to gum tissue (occlusal traumatism). Teeth bordering on empty spaces can drift and rotate: food can collect, cavities may develop, and eventually periodontal disease can result. To prevent this or to correct it before extensive damage is done, minor surgery or braces (orthodontic correction) may be recommended.

Any abnormal force exerted by the tongue, lips, or cheek muscles against the teeth can also result in damage to gum tissue. Treatment involves learning to speak, breathe, and swallow properly to alleviate any unnecessary pressure on your teeth and gums.

Bruxism, the habit of grinding or clenching your teeth, can also contribute to the development of periodontal disease. Most sufferers of bruxism grind their teeth while sleeping; treatment may involve the use of a plastic mouth guard fitted over the upper or lower teeth.

Poor tooth alignment

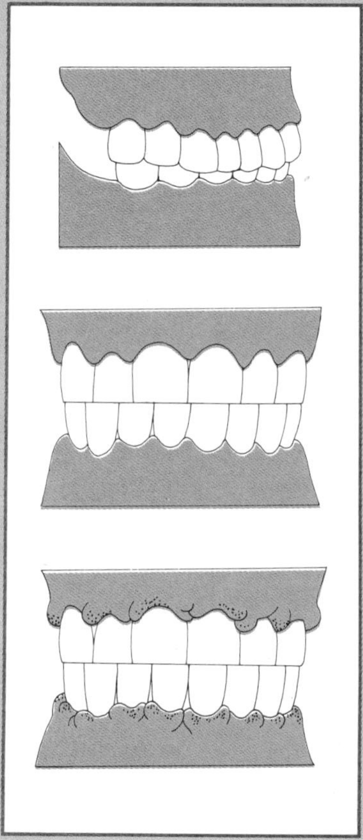

Overbite...

or tooth grinding(bruxism)...

can lead to gum disease.

The Keyes technique

The Keyes technique, or modulated and monitored therapy, is a nonsurgical treatment for periodontal disease. (This technique's named for a dentist and former research scientist with the National Institute of Dental Research.) The treatment calls for close monitoring of your mouth's bacteria by your dentist and a rigorous program for you of at-home oral hygiene.

The at-home program involves daily brushing with a solution of baking soda, salt, and hydrogen peroxide; flossing; and using a warm, saltwater solution with an oral irrigation device. Antibiotics are sometimes prescribed.

The Keyes technique, a conservative approach to periodontal disease, is controversial because it doesn't enable you to reach any bacteria working under the gum's surface. The American Academy of Periodontology has stated that while the Keyes technique is an excellent form of prevention, it doesn't eliminate the need for periodontal surgery in advanced cases.

Prevention of periodontal disease

None of the treatments for periodontal disease is pleasant, and they can all be expensive and time-consuming. Since periodontal disease is the result of neglect, the best treatment is prevention. The ADA sums it up best in this motto: "Ignore your teeth and they'll go away."

The same steps you take to prevent tooth decay serve to prevent gum disease. Use disclosing tablets occasionally to make sure you're removing all the plaque, and pay special attention to your gums and the base of your teeth when brushing and flossing. And remember that no matter how carefully you care for your teeth, you'll also need regular dental checkups.

6 Using a Specialist

What is pulp?
The tooth pulp contains nerves, connective tissue, and blood vessels and is essential to a tooth's life because it provides necessary nutrients to the dentin.

Your dentist can treat you for all routine dental problems and the early stages of periodontal disease. However, you may develop a dental problem that requires treatment by a specialist. For example, if you have a serious gum disease, you'll need to see a periodontist. Following are other dental specialists and the conditions they treat.

Endodontist

An endodontist specializes in the diagnosis and treatment of tooth pulp diseases. If the tooth's pulp is damaged—for example, from a blow to your jaw, a broken or fractured tooth, or advanced periodontal disease—an infection can occur, causing an abscess. An abscess can also result from tooth decay that has spread to a tooth's nerve. To save the affected tooth, you may need a root canal.

Pain is your signal that the pulp has been affected. The severity and duration of the pain indicate the amount of damage. Pain that results from an abscess will be severe. You may also have a fever, and the side of your face may swell. You should see your dentist or an endodontist.

If the abscess results from periodontal disease, the nerve is still alive. The endodontist will drain the abscessed gum tissue and clean your teeth carefully.

If the abscess results from tooth decay, the tooth's nerve is dying. Your endodontist will open the tooth and drain the abscess and probably prescribe antibiotics to prevent the infection from spreading.

If you need a root canal, the endodontist will test the nerve to see if it's still functioning. If it isn't, then he'll remove the nerve. The endodontist will clean out the root canal in preparation for a filling. He'll smooth and wash the root canal with a germicidal solution to remove any remaining bacteria. Then he'll dry, medicate, and temporarily seal the canal.

When you return for your next appointment, the endodontist will check for bacteria. If no bacteria are present, the endodontist will seal the canal with a rubberlike substance to prevent bacteria from entering the canal. Since your tooth no longer has a nerve, it will need reinforcement with a pin. A crown can then protect what remains of the tooth.

In addition to the standard root canal treatment, the endodontist may need to use surgical endodontics to reach the diseased areas. In apical curettage, the endodontist makes an incision in the gum to get to the abscessed area and then scrapes out the affected tissues surrounding the root. An apicoectomy involves cutting away a portion of the root tip.

Root canal treatment usually requires two to four appointments, depending on the case's severity.

What happens in a root canal

To prepare a tooth for root canal therapy, the endodontist drills through the crown of the tooth into the pulp chamber. He then inserts endodontic instruments into the canals to file and ream the canals clean in preparation for sealing.

Root canal

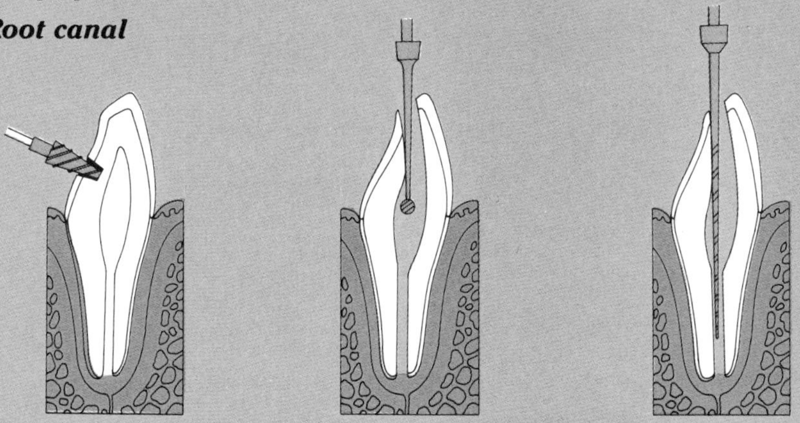

Drilling through the crown ***Drilling into pulp*** ***Cleaning out the canal***

Apicoectomy

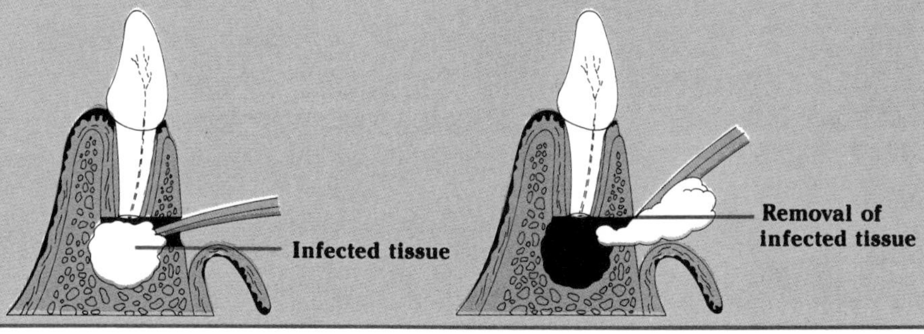

Women and TMJ
Eighty percent of the people treated for TMJ are women, usually in their twenties or thirties.

Temporomandibular joint syndrome

Temporomandibular joint syndrome (TMJ) is a disorder of the joint between the jaw and cheekbone that causes limited jaw movement, pain (particularly around the ear), and a clicking or popping sound when you move your jaw. TMJ results from undue stress on the temporomandibular joint. This joint connects the upper and lower jaw and, together with five pairs of muscles and several ligaments, helps you chew and speak.

Several factors can bring on TMJ, among them old age and the accompanying lack of muscle tone, arthritis, a blow to the head, and teeth that don't fit together properly. Bad habits like gum chewing, nail biting, jaw jutting, or cheek and lip chewing can also cause undue stress on the temporomandibular area. However, the most common cause of this disorder is teeth grinding or clenching (bruxism), usually due to stress.

TMJ can cause symptoms that seem to be unrelated to your mouth, such as neck or shoulder pains, earaches, ringing in the ears, and dizziness. The most common symptoms are severe facial pain and clicking and popping sounds when you open and close your mouth.

Research on TMJ is under way, but no professional consensus exists on its treatment. Sometimes the cure is as simple as stopping bad habits like nail biting or gum chewing. If the cause of the problem is tooth grinding or clenching, a mouth guard worn at night may bring relief. Muscle relaxants can promote relaxation of the involved face and neck muscles. Some people respond well to biofeedback techniques.

If poorly aligned teeth are the problem, your dentist may grind some tooth surfaces to redistribute stress in your jaw or suggest orthodontia.

Ten to 15% of TMJ patients require surgery. Several clinics in the United States currently treat patients with TMJ. To get information on clinics near you, contact the American Dental Association, 211 East Chicago Avenue, Chicago, IL 60611 (312-440-2500).

The area affected by TMJ

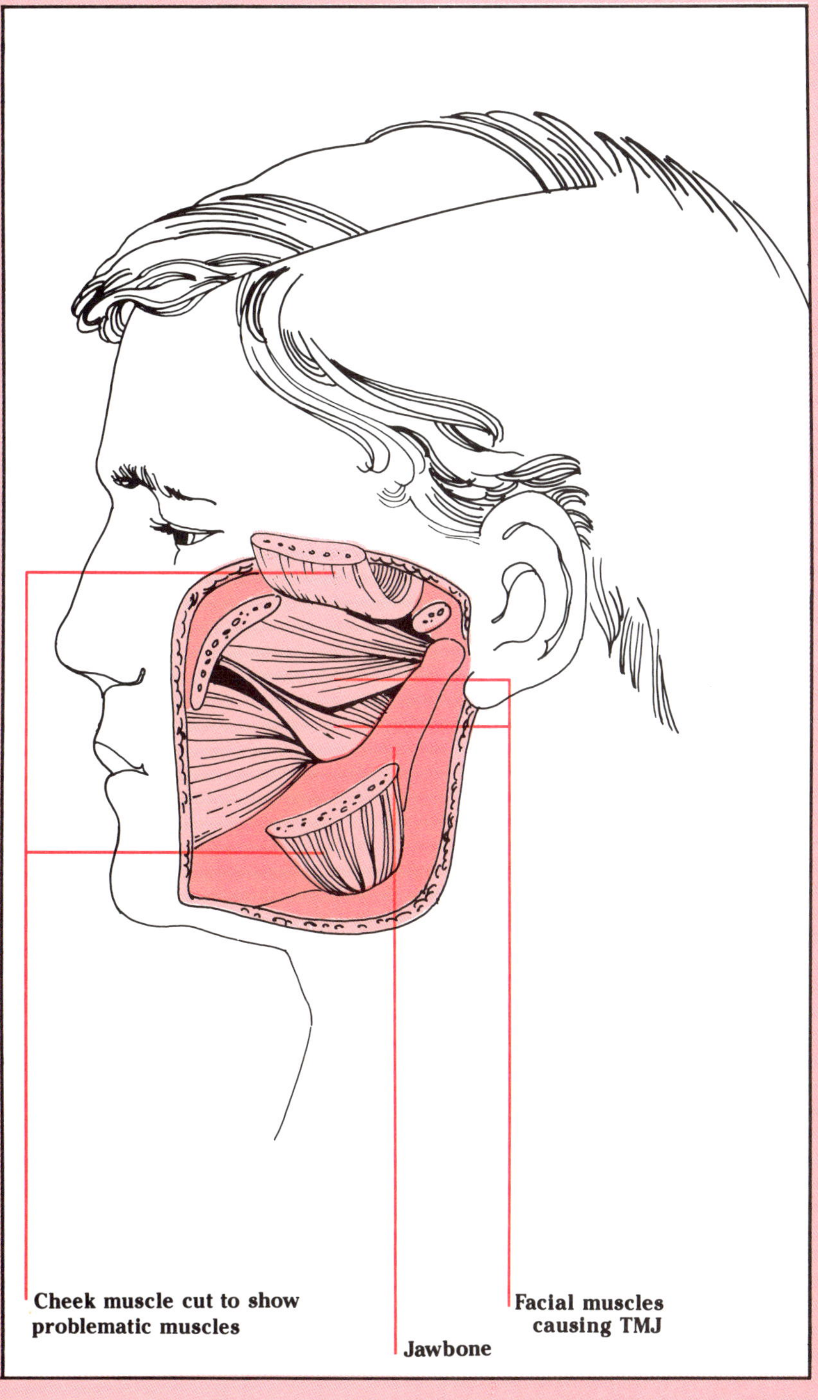

Other gum problems

Besides performing gum flap surgery, a periodontist can use gingivectomy to cut away excess gum tissue for cosmetic purposes. He can reshape gum tissue to improve its fit around teeth—a process called gingivoplasty. And he can perform gum grafting—surgically moving small amounts of gum from one part of the mouth to another.

Periodontist

A periodontist specializes in diseases of the gums and supporting tissue. He'll perform periodontal therapy and surgery, if necessary. This surgery removes calculus from the deep pockets that have formed. It may also involve making the pockets smaller and reshaping the gum tissue so that you can more easily clean your teeth under the gumline.

Various types of periodontal surgery can help restore gum tissue to a healthy state. A periodontist selects the type appropriate for the extent of the gum disease.

If pockets have formed but the bone hasn't been affected, the periodontist may select a surgical procedure known as gingivectomy. This procedure removes the soft gum tissue that forms the wall of the pocket. Your periodontist will probably trim and reshape the gumline after he's eliminated the pockets. If only a few teeth are affected, you may need one visit only. However, if the damage is extensive, you'll need several appointments because your periodontist will treat your mouth in sections.

If the pockets are too deep for effective gingivectomy or if the bone has been affected, the periodontist may perform *flap surgery.* In this procedure, the periodontist cuts the affected gum tissue to form a flap that he can fold out and reach the tooth's root. Once the periodontist has access to the tooth's root, he'll remove any calculus, plaque, and diseased tissue. He'll then sew (suture) your gum back into position. This procedure may include bone reconstructing and contouring (osseous resection).

If the underlying damage is extensive, you may need to have the affected teeth extracted. Remaining teeth can be joined together with screws and metal pins that provide stability and support. If all the teeth are undermined, you'll lose them and have to wear dentures.

Two gum treatments

Gingivectomy

In gingivectomy, a thin ribbon of gingival tissue is surgically removed to eliminate gum pockets caused by early-stage periodontal disease.

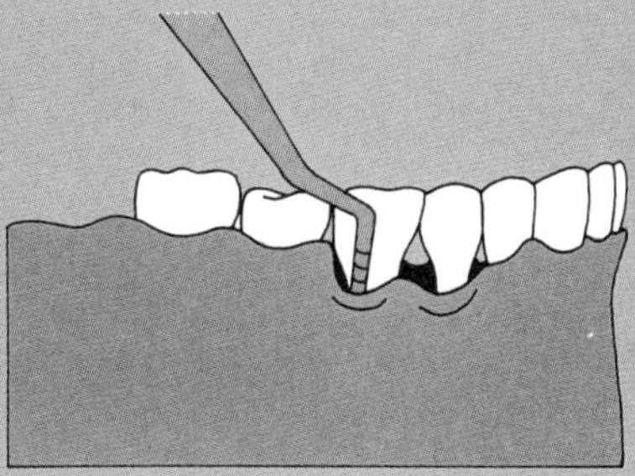

Removing a thin layer of gum tissue

Flap surgery

If periodontal disease is advanced and bony pockets are present, flap surgery may be necessary. In this procedure, incisions in the gum create a flap that can be pulled away from the teeth roots, enabling the specialist to remove diseased tissue and, if necessary, reshape the bone.

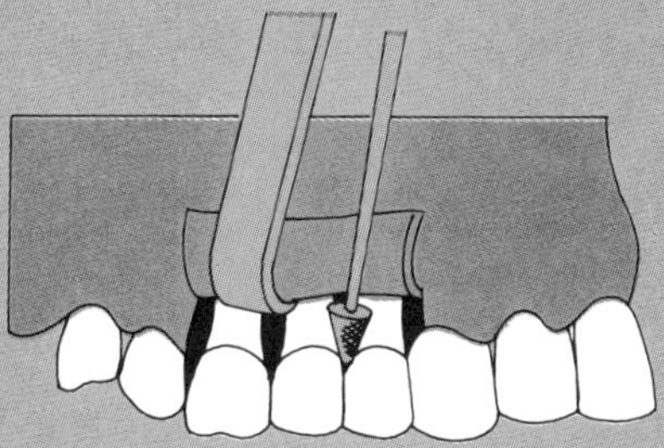

Flap surgery and removal of diseased tissue

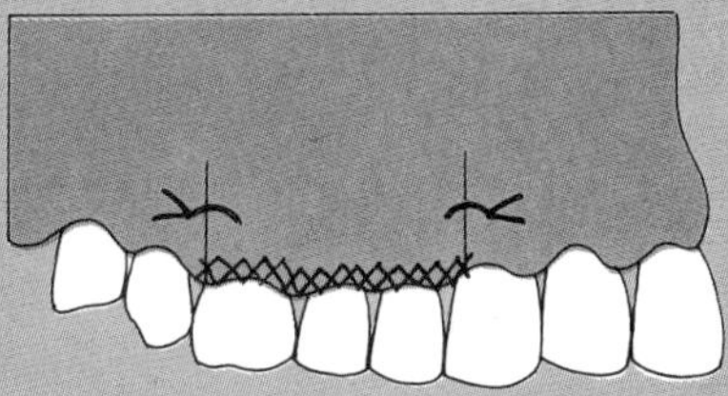

Gum stitched into place after surgery

Other surgery

An oral surgeon can reshape a jaw to correct poor bites. He'll use drills, saws, or chisels to cut and rearrange bones to correct a protruding lower jaw, a bite where teeth don't meet, or an upper lip that too greatly hides the upper teeth. Usually, he'll work from within the mouth, leaving no outside scars or markings.

Oral surgeon

An oral surgeon specializes in surgical procedures in the mouth. The most likely reason for you to visit an oral surgeon is to have your wisdom teeth removed.

Wisdom teeth are the last teeth in the back of each group of molars. Most people get their four wisdom teeth between the ages of 17 and 21. Sometimes one or more of the wisdom teeth never emerge, sometimes they emerge at an angle, sometimes they're diseased, and sometimes they become blocked (impacted) under the gum.

If a wisdom tooth doesn't emerge, you'll probably suffer no symptoms. However, a wisdom tooth that emerges at an angle or becomes impacted can cause problems. Gum tissue surrounding a partially erupted or impacted wisdom tooth may become inflamed and infected: you'll need to have the wisdom tooth removed surgically. Your dentist may perform this operation or may refer you to an oral surgeon. If the wisdom tooth is positioned at a difficult angle or if other wisdom teeth present problems and must be removed at the same time, you may need to be hospitalized briefly.

The oral surgeon may use either a local or a general anesthetic. To remove the wisdom tooth, the oral surgeon may have to cut the tooth into sections. After removing the tooth, the surgeon will clean out any remaining tooth chips or bone fragments. The opening is then cleaned thoroughly and surgically closed. Most people experience some pain and swelling for a few days after the procedure, and the oral surgeon may prescribe medication for the pain. Contact the oral surgeon if the pain persists.

Impacted wisdom teeth

Wisdom teeth are the teeth most frequently impacted. A widsom tooth becomes impacted when no room remains for it to erupt through the gum into the mouth. An impaction is partial when a portion of the tooth's crown has protruded through the gum; full, when no part of the tooth protrudes. An impacted wisdom tooth is susceptible to infection and cyst formation and can also affect adjacent teeth, exposing them to infection and possibly moving them out of proper alignment.

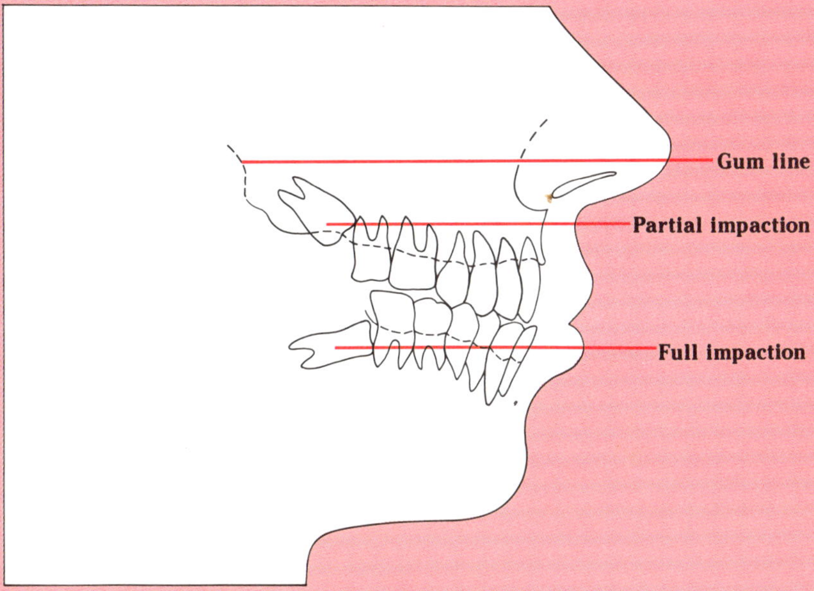

Oral symptoms
Some illnesses—among them scarlet fever, diphtheria, measles, tuberculosis, and gonorrhea—can be identified by their effects on the mouth.

Oral pathologist

An oral pathologist specializes in the diagnosis and treatment of diseases that affect the teeth, jawbones, tongue, lips, and salivary glands. These diseases include everything from plaque and common gingivitis to oral syphilis and cancer.

If you have a viral infection in your mouth, your dentist or doctor may refer you to an oral pathologist. The most common oral virus is herpes simplex, which causes cold sores on your lips and on the inside of your mouth. This virus seems to affect adolescents and young adults more frequently than adults, but some people suffer regularly from cold sores.

Herpes simplex of the mouth is common and rarely serious. The sores usually disappear by themselves in 2 to 3 weeks. The recommended home care treatment is to place ice wrapped in a cloth directly on the spot at the onset of the sores (this treatment isn't effective after the sores have developed). If the sores are severe, your doctor or dentist may prescribe a corticosteroid cream or antiviral agent for you to apply to the sores.

Mouth ulcers, including canker sores, are relatively common. Most mouth ulcers appear on the lining of your lips, cheek, and tongue. They can appear in clusters or individually and can be painful enough to interfere with normal mouth movements, such as talking, chewing, or swallowing. Mouth ulcers usually heal within 5 to 14 days and rarely scar.

The exact cause of mouth ulcers isn't known. Allergies, stress, heredity, drugs, and poor diet have all been suggested as possible causes. Some people seem to have a tendency to develop them and do so repeatedly.

No single treatment is effective for everyone, but you may find one of the following suggestions helpful. If the ulcers are so painful that they interfere with eating, you may want to try a mild topical anesthetic liquid and apply it before meals. Oral antihistamines used before you eat and at bedtime may offer relief. Some dental professionals recommend drinking a glass of water with 10 drops of diluted hydrochloric acid (10%—no stronger) once a day until the ulcers heal.

Oral pathologists also treat fungal and bacterial infections of the mouth and vitamin deficiencies that affect the mouth (such deficiencies are rare in the United States).

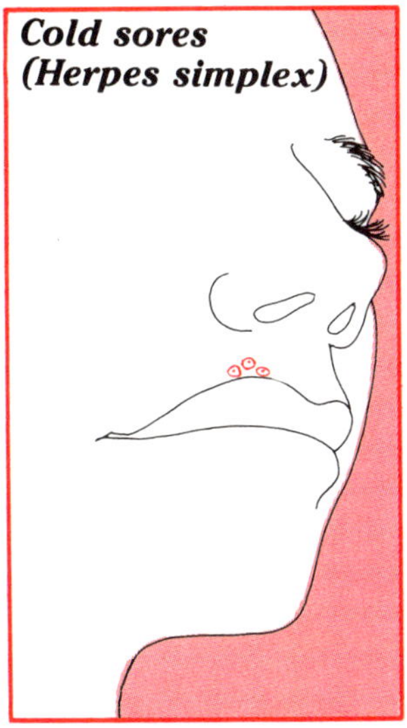

Cold sores (Herpes simplex)

Tumors can occur anywhere in your mouth. The causes of these tumors aren't known exactly, but excessive smoking and alcohol consumption may be contributing factors. Such tumors may be either benign or malignant. A benign tumor doesn't spread and isn't life-threatening; a malignant tumor is cancer that may spread.

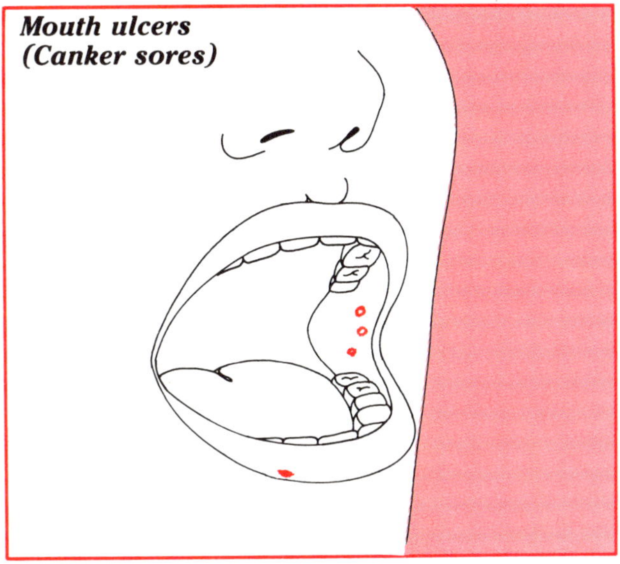

Mouth ulcers (Canker sores)

Mouth diseases

During your regular checkup, your dentist will examine your teeth for signs of decay and your gums for signs of gum disease. Your dentist will also examine the lining of your mouth for signs of mouth disease. Although many of these diseases have nothing to do with your teeth, your dentist is in a good position to detect such diseases in their early stages.

You, too, should be alert to any color or texture changes in your mouth's lining. Most mouth diseases aren't serious and are easy to treat, but you should always consult your dentist or doctor if you think you have a mouth disease or a mouth tumor. Here are some of the mouth diseases your dentist will look for:

• ***Oral thrush.*** Various fungi are present in your mouth at all times. Under certain circumstances—such as when your resistance to infection is low after you've been ill or when a course of treatment with antibiotics has upset the natural balance among the microorganisms in your mouth—some of these fungi

(text continued on page 72)

Self-examination for oral tumors

Your dentist may examine your mouth for signs of tumors during your regular checkup. You should examine your mouth yourself at least once every 6 months. Follow these steps:

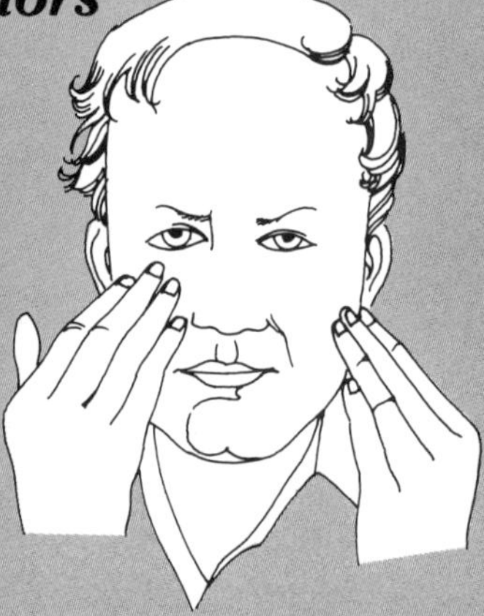

1. Check for any new lumps, bumps, or signs of swelling on your face.

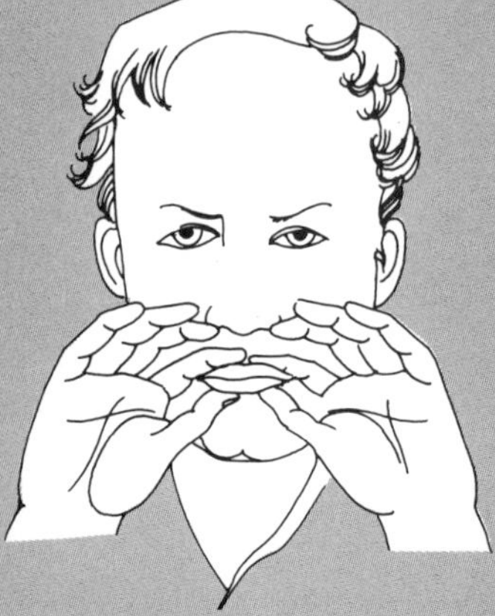

2. Press your lips together. Do you feel any lip lumps? Has the outline of your mouth changed in any way?

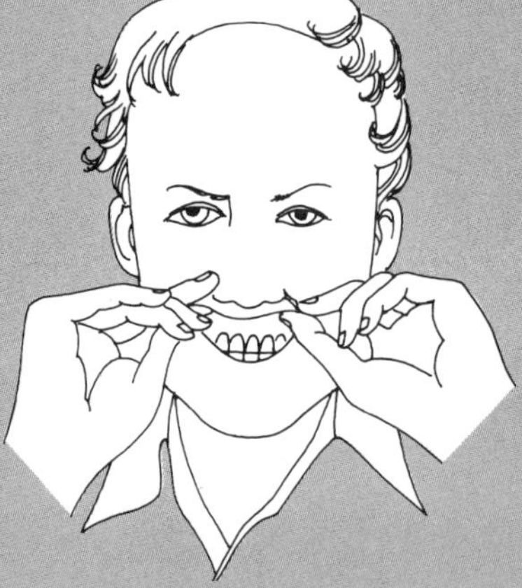

3. Check your gums for new lumps, bumps, or signs of swelling. Check for ulcers or swollen areas that won't heal. Check for any white patches.

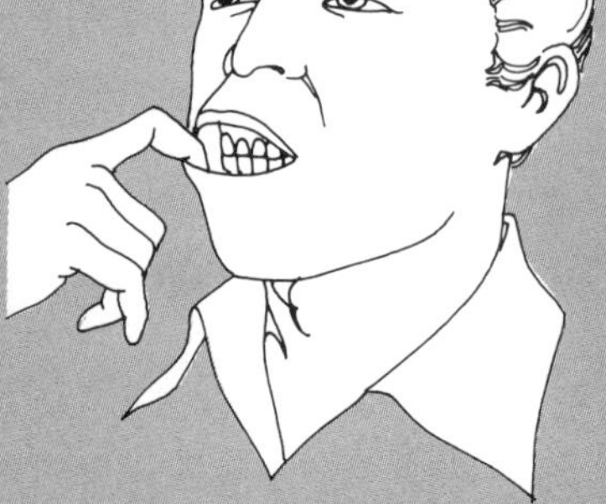

4. Feel the inside of your cheeks for any rough spots, lumps, or bumps. Use a mirror to examine the inside of your cheeks for white spots or color changes.

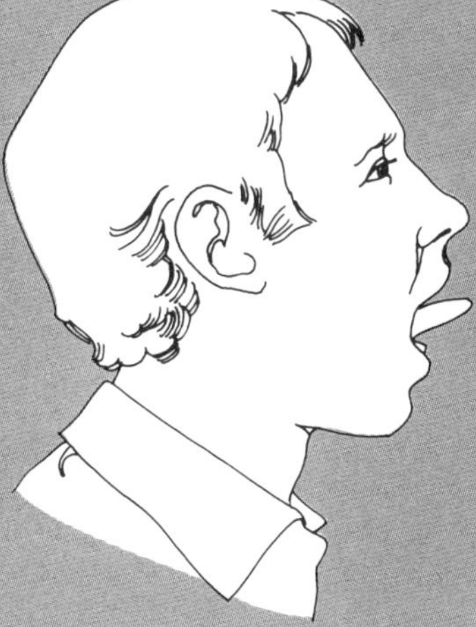

5. Examine the surface of your tongue and the roof of your mouth for any lumps, bumps, color changes, sore spots, or ulcers.

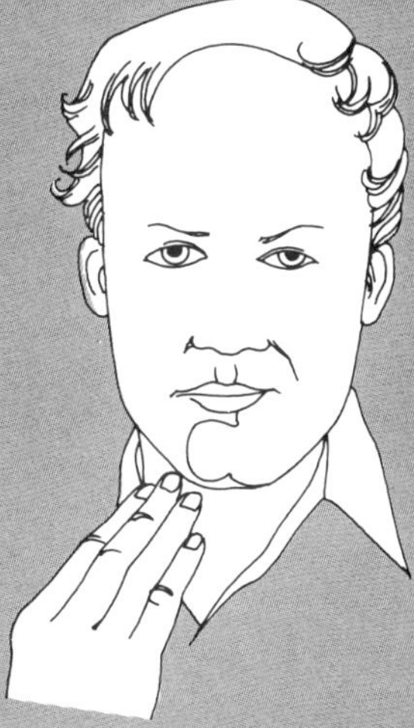

6. Feel the sides of your neck for any swellings.

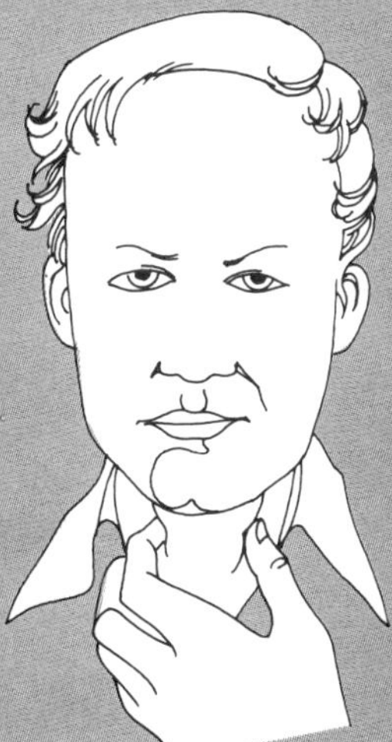

7. Put your fingers on your Adam's apple. It should rise when you swallow. Check for unusual lumps or bumps as you swallow.

See your doctor immediately if you notice something unusual. Also see your doctor or dentist immediately if your dentures have begun to fit badly, if your tongue has become stiff and hard to control, or if you have any prolonged hoarseness not from an ordinary cold or sore throat.

can multiply. Oral thrush results from the uncontrolled growth of the *Candida albicans* fungus. The signs of oral thrush are sore patches in your mouth and, sometimes, down your throat. The patches are milky yellow and slightly raised.

Most common in young children and the elderly, oral thrush isn't serious and can be successfully treated with medicines. However, oral thrush tends to recur.

• ***Oral lichen planus.*** This disease involves changes in your mouth's soft, delicate lining. The disease usually begins as a group of small pimples that, with time, join to form a network of thin, gray, lacy ridges. Or the disease may appear as shiny, red, slightly raised patches. These symptoms occur on the inside of your cheeks and the sides of your tongue. In addition, you may sense mouth soreness and have a dry, metallic taste.

This rare disease's causes aren't known, but emotional stress, mouth irritation such as that caused by ill-fitting dentures, and poor oral hygiene are probably contributing factors. Your dentist can treat this disease with drugs.

• ***Leukoplakia.*** This disease involves a thickening and hardening of part of the normally soft lining of your mouth. This usually results from soreness or irritation caused by ill-fitting dentures or a rough tooth; the heat of inhaled tobacco smoke can also cause this reaction. The thickening and hardening are actually your mouth's method of protecting the delicate skin.

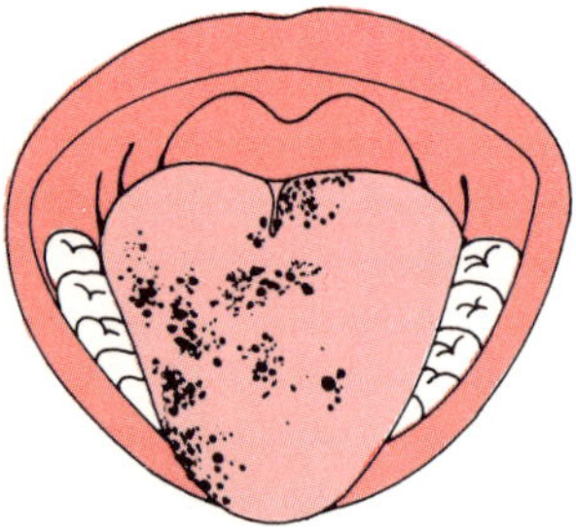

Hardened skin patches on tongue

With time, the hardened skin patch may become white or gray; although such patches rarely cause discomfort when they begin growing, they eventually feel rough and may be sensitive to hot or spicy foods.

The best treatment for leukoplakia is removal of the irritation. This can mean having your dentures refitted, having a tooth smoothed down, or giving up smoking. Irritant elimination usually solves the problem, but your dentist may decide to take a biopsy of the patch—he'll remove a small portion and send it to a laboratory for testing. A biopsy is sensible because leukoplakia can be an early sign of mouth cancer.

Thumb sucking and buck teeth

Most dentists believe that buck teeth are the result of heredity, not thumb sucking. Although a child's baby teeth may be affected by constant thumb sucking, permanent teeth won't be harmed unless the habit continues past about age 4.

Pedodontist

A pedodontist specializes in dentistry for children. At-home dental care for children should begin even before a child's first tooth emerges. By age 2, most children have all of their 20 primary teeth—this is the time for the child's first visit to the dentist.

The pedodontist treats children's dental problems but also educates parents. Many parents believe tooth decay and dental problems are inevitable parts of aging. They aren't, of course, and pedodontists stress the importance of proper care of baby teeth.

Baby bottle syndrome and other dental concerns

Bottle feeding is the leading source of dental problems for children under age 3. Most fruit juices and formulas may contain sugar; milk contains lactose, a form of sugar, and other carbohydrates that feed mouth bacteria. The most common sign of this syndrome is badly decayed upper front teeth—the bottle's nipple rests just behind these teeth when the child sucks.

If your child has already developed the habit of going to bed with a bottle of milk or juice, gradually reduce the amount of sugary liquid by diluting it with water. Continue diluting the liquid until the bottle contains only water.

Thumb or finger sucking is common among children and rarely presents a problem. Most children stop sucking their thumbs around age 2; if they continue to suck their thumbs past about age 4, however, it can affect the shape of the child's jawbone and the alignment of the teeth. If your child still sucks a thumb beyond age 4, you'll need professional help for that habit. Consult your dentist.

If your child loses a primary tooth from an accident or extraction and the space isn't filled while you're waiting for the permanent tooth to erupt, his other teeth may drift. To prevent this, a pedodontist will fit a maintainer for the space. The same procedure is performed for older children with missing teeth.

How milk bathes the front teeth

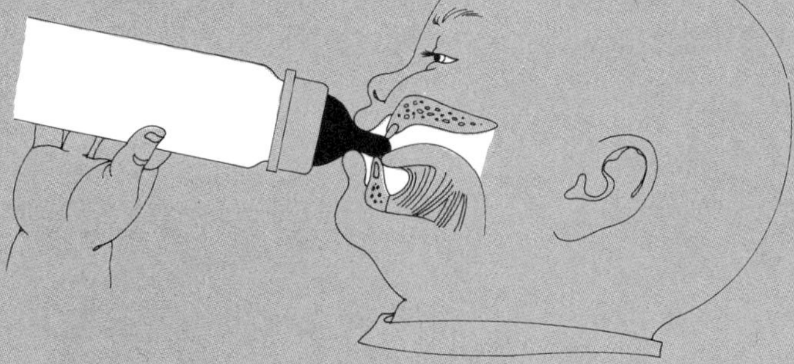

How to tell if your child needs orthodontic work

If any of the following conditions exists in the mouth of an 8-year-old or older child, arrange a consultation with your dentist:

- front teeth irregularity—overlapping; teeth turned in, out, sideways; one tooth noticeably longer or shorter than the others
- top teeth cover bottom teeth completely when the back teeth are in contact
- front teeth spaces
- a gap between the top and bottom front teeth when the back teeth are in contact (overbite)
- lower front teeth extend over upper front teeth when the back teeth are in contact.

Ask yourself these questions about your child's appearance:

- Does the child have a receding chin?
- Do the child's lips bulge because of protruding teeth or does the child's bite close differently on one side than on the other?
- When the child opens or closes the mouth, does the jaw move straight up and down, or does it swing to one side only?

Identifying bad oral habits in children

Thumb sucking is recognized by parents as a bad habit that can contribute to malocclusion. If your child sucks his thumb, consult your dentist for advice on when and how to deal with the habit. Lip, finger, and nail biting and pushing the tongue against the teeth when swallowing can also contribute to malocclusion. Look for the following signs of bad oral habits and work with your child to correct them.

Habit	***Signs***
Biting lips	*Chapped lips, swollen lower lip, bleeding lips*
Pushing tongue against front teeth when swallowing	*Chin muscles wrinkle when child swallows*
Biting fingernails	*Short fingernails*
Chewing cheeks	*Swollen and inflamed areas inside of cheeks*
Biting fingers	*Calluses on fingers; ragged skin around nails*
Thumb sucking	*Wrinkled and clean thumb*

Prosthodontist

A prosthodontist specializes in the replacement of missing teeth by bridges or dentures. If you lose a tooth or teeth or have one or more teeth extracted, you'll need to have a bridge or partial denture made to prevent your remaining teeth from shifting. If you lose all your teeth, you'll need full dentures.

Orthodontist

An orthodontist specializes in the diagnosis, prevention, and treatment of crooked, separated, or improperly aligned teeth. This sometimes involves correcting underslung or protruding jaws. Orthodontic work is rarely only cosmetic; properly aligned teeth are less prone to cavities and periodontal disease.

Improperly aligned teeth are usually inherited—a condition known as inherited malocclusion. However, improperly aligned teeth can also be brought on by neglect, bad oral habits, or disease—known as acquired malocclusion.

Braces

Braces must be fit carefully. The orthodontist will examine and X-ray your child's teeth and make a plaster cast of the teeth, gums, and jaws. The orthodontist may also take measurements and photographs of your child's face.

After he's planned a treatment program, the orthodontist will fit the child with the braces. Over a period of time, the orthodontist will adjust brackets on the braces to gradually move individual teeth into the desired position. Braces cause discomfort, when they're first put in place and when they're adjusted.

Oral hygiene is extremely important during this period, and the child should brush, floss, and use an oral irrigation device even though doing so may be quite uncomfortable. Continued regular visits to the

Children and adolescents

Improper tooth alignment (malocclusion) becomes noticeable in children when their permanent teeth first begin to erupt. If your child is seeing a pedodontist regularly, the pedodontist will spot the malocclusion early and may then refer you to an orthodontist.

Malocclusions are divided into three general classes: two refer to overbites; the third to an underbite. Orthodontic appliances that apply pressure can correct malocclusions by moving teeth into proper positions. These appliances are best known as braces.

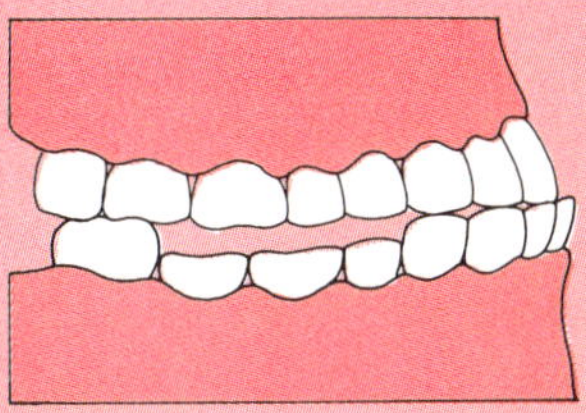

Underbite

Keeping teeth apart

The ends of our teeth aren't meant to touch for more than about 90 minutes each day. Except for those moments of actual tooth contact, when you're talking or chewing, your facial muscles should be at rest, leaving a gap of from 1 to 2 mm between your upper and lower teeth.

dentist are necessary to catch any decay during its initial stage.

If your child has bands that fit around each tooth, he'll need to see the orthodontist as soon as possible whenever a band loosens. Loose bands allow food to collect, which can cause decay.

Orthodontic treatment can last 2 or more years. When the braces are removed, a retainer may be used. If teeth have been moved too quickly, new bone supporting the teeth in their new positions may not have enough time to form. The retainer is usually used at night for gradually decreasing periods until it's no longer necessary.

New options in braces

While conventional metal band braces are still widely used, you now have the option of wearing several different kinds of less visible braces that are held in place with bonding glues.

How teeth are moved

Teeth are set in bone, and bone can be remolded by pressure. If you wear braces, the wires and elastic bands (or small springs) apply pressure to the teeth and bones. When a tooth's under pressure, the tooth root pushes on the surrounding bone. The bone softens in the pressured area and the tooth moves into this softened space. After the tooth moves, new bone forms to hold the tooth in its new position.

- Lingual braces are brackets and wires bonded to the inner side (lingual, or tongue, side) of the teeth. The biggest advantage to lingual braces is appearance, since they're hidden behind the teeth. Lingual braces are difficult to fit and often cost more than other types of braces. They can cause tongue irritation and a speech impediment because the distance between the tongue and the teeth is reduced.
- Clear plastic braces are brackets that hold wires on the front of the teeth and are less obvious than conventional metal braces. Clear plastic braces are best if you need only minor orthodontic work. The plastic may become stained and is easily broken, so you'll need special care when you eat and clean your teeth. The cost and treatment time for plastic braces are similar to those for metal braces. Some dentists will use clear plastic braces on upper teeth and metal braces on the lowers, for appearance.
- Ceramic braces are also less conspicuous than metal braces because they're your teeth's color. Problems with ceramic braces include stains, difficult fit with metal wires, and brittleness.
- Metal-mesh brackets are another choice. The brackets are glued to the teeth surfaces, eliminating the need for conventional braces' metal rings. These brackets are small and unobtrusive, but they're just as effective as metal bands.

Three types of braces

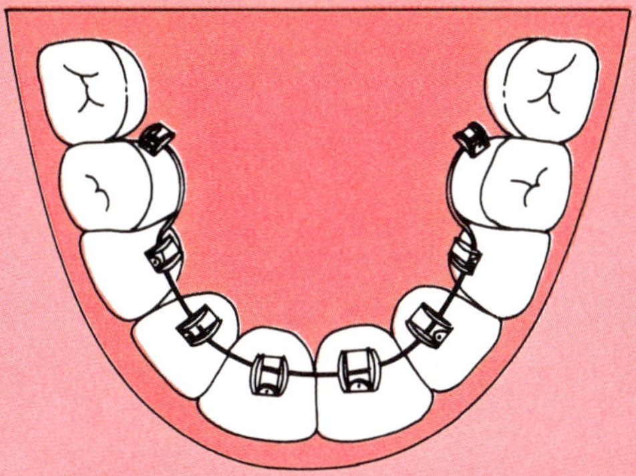

Lingual braces

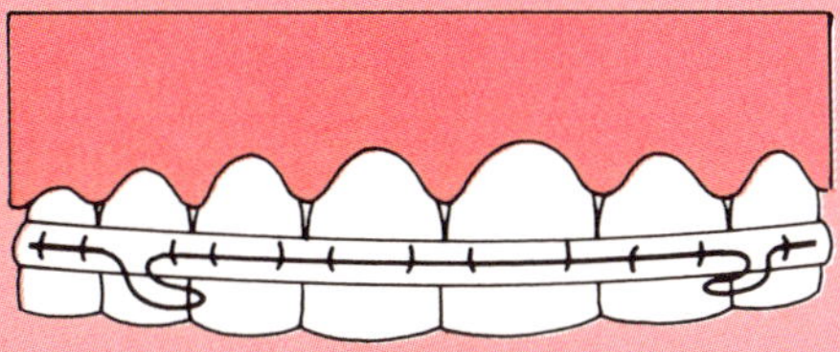

Clear plastic braces

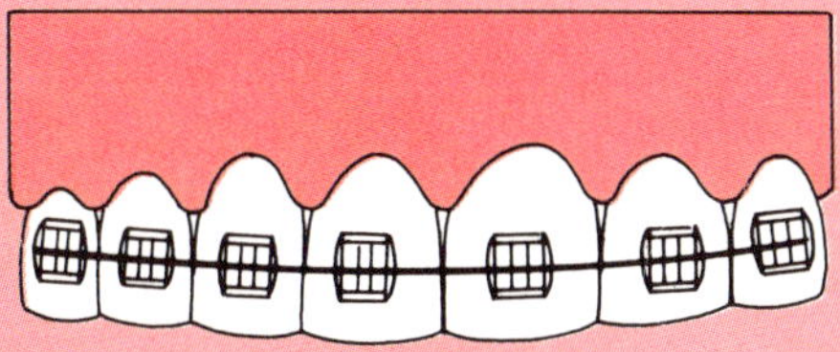

Metal-mesh brackets

Adults

More adults seek orthodontic treatment today than in the past. Some are getting treatment their families couldn't afford; others are having their teeth straightened for a more comfortable bite or to prevent possible periodontal problems.

However, orthodontic treatment for adults poses special problems. Because an adult's jaws and teeth have almost stopped growing, orthodontic treatment can take longer. An adult's teeth can't be moved as far or as easily as a child's. The chance is also greater that the teeth will shift back into their original position once the appliance has been removed.

Although orthodontic treatment can be expensive, it can save you money in the long run by saving the health of your teeth. Orthodontia may mean fewer later problems that can lead to root canals and bridges.

7

Wearing a Bridge

Dental bridges can be divided into two categories: fixed bridges and removable ones.

Once put in position, a fixed bridge can't be removed. The teeth on either side of the space to be filled provide support for the bridge. These healthy teeth are usually covered with crowns to which the bridge is attached. As long as the supporting teeth on either side of a space are healthy and strong, a fixed bridge can replace most of the teeth on either the upper or lower jaw.

A cantilevered bridge uses only one healthy tooth as support. While neither as stable nor as strong as a fixed bridge that's attached on either side, a cantilevered bridge is often used on the last back tooth or, for cosmetic purposes, on front teeth. The strength of a cantilevered bridge depends on the health of the supporting tooth.

At first, a new bridge may feel bulky and awkward, and the pressure put on the teeth to which the bridge is anchored can cause soreness. This discomfort may last quite a while. However, you'll eventually adjust to the bridge and no longer notice its presence.

Cleaning around a bridge requires a little extra attention. Regardless of how well a bridge is constructed, food particles can become trapped in it. Use the same soft toothbrush you use for your normal teeth, and scrub the tops and sides of the bridge. Remember to brush your gums to increase the blood circulation. Then floss thoroughly.

Removable bridge

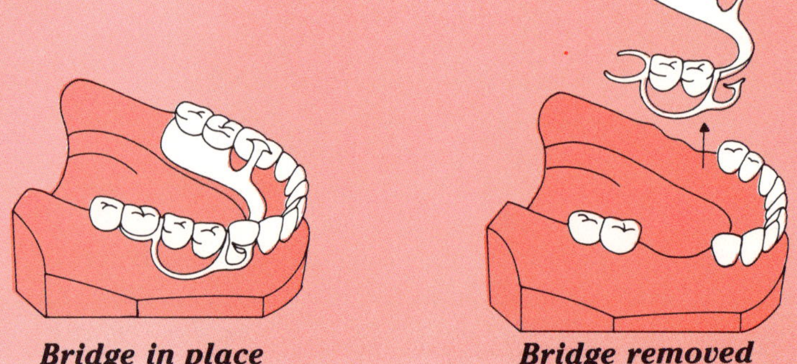

Bridge in place ***Bridge removed***

Types of fixed bridges

To replace a missing tooth with a conventional fixed bridge, one tooth on either side of the missing tooth is prepared to receive the bridge. Then the bridge—usually porcelain fused to a metal framework—is fitted over the prepared teeth and just under the gum tissue.

If you have sound teeth on just one side of the missing tooth, you might need a cantilevered bridge. This type of bridge is anchored on one side only to one or more teeth and is suspended over the gap left by the missing tooth.

Cantilevered bridge

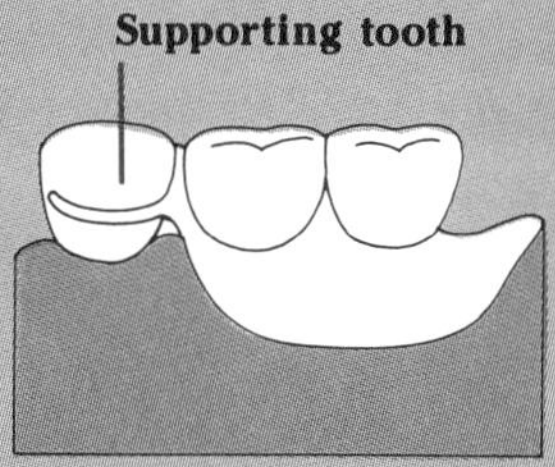

Conventional fixed bridge

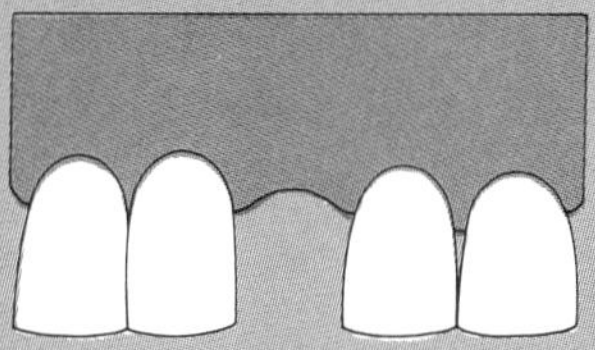

Missing tooth

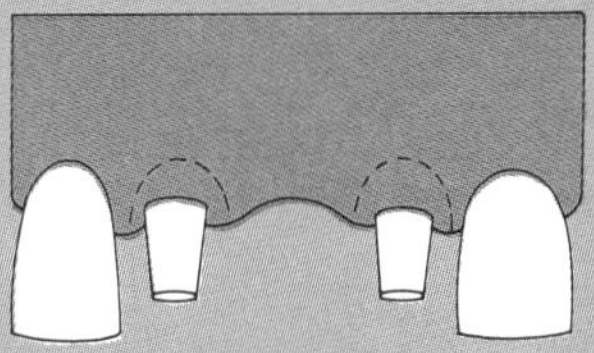

One tooth on either side of missing tooth is drilled into a post shape.

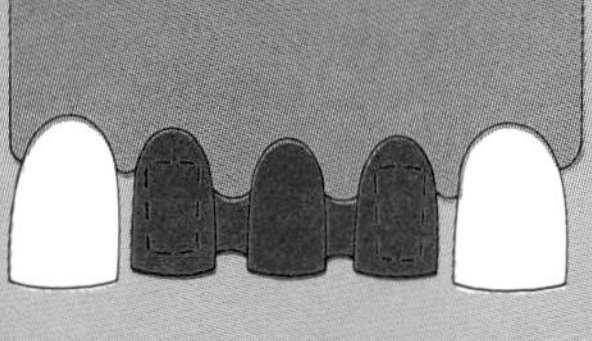

Metal framework in position

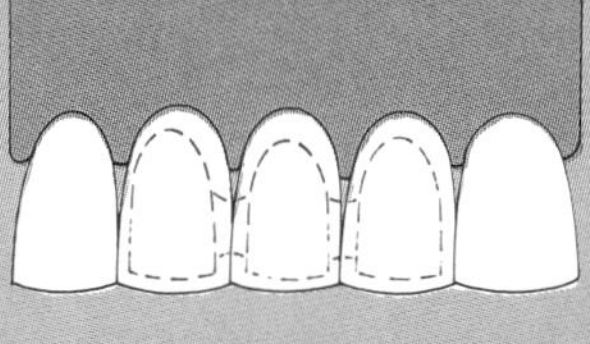

Final porcelain-covered bridge in position

How to floss around a bridge

To floss around a bridge, you'll need a special flexible threader. Follow these steps:

Place about 18 to 20 inches of floss through the threader.

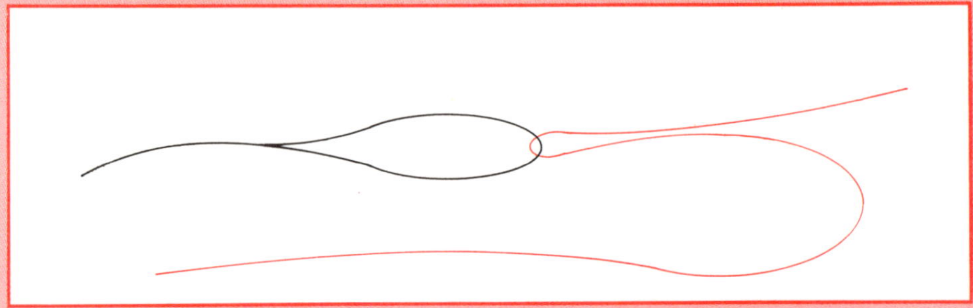

Carefully push the threader's straight end through the space between the bridge and each supporting tooth.

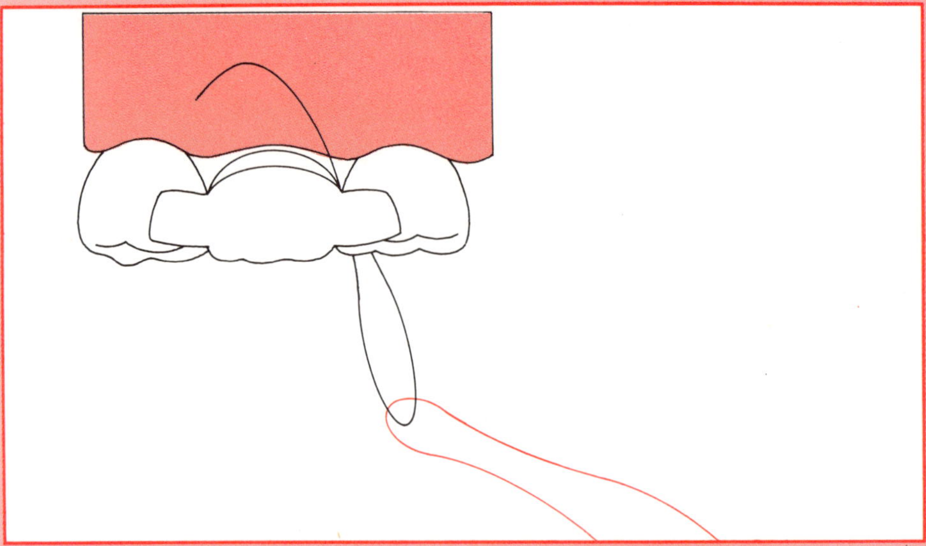

Then pull the threader and floss through, remove the threader from the floss, and hold both ends of the floss.

Move the floss gently between the gum tissue and the artificial tooth to clean beneath the gum and the bridge.

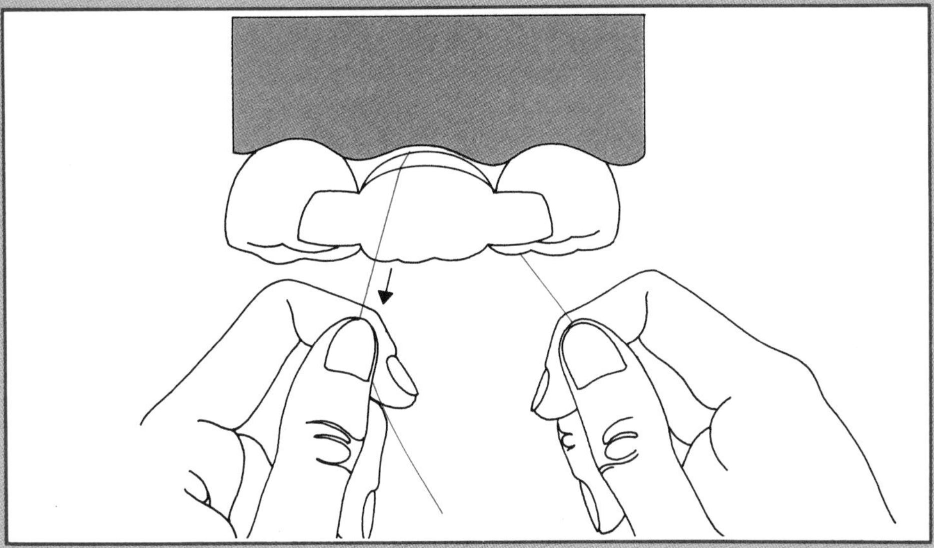

Move the floss against the side of one of the supporting teeth; move it up and down to clean the side.

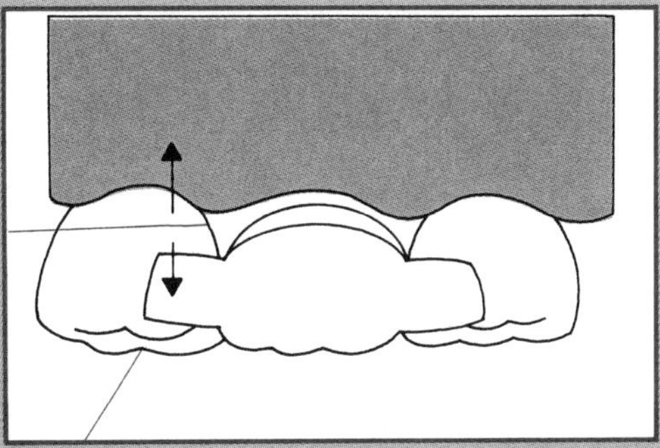

Guide the floss between the gum tissue and the artificial tooth next to the other supporting tooth.

Repeat the flossing procedure; rinse.

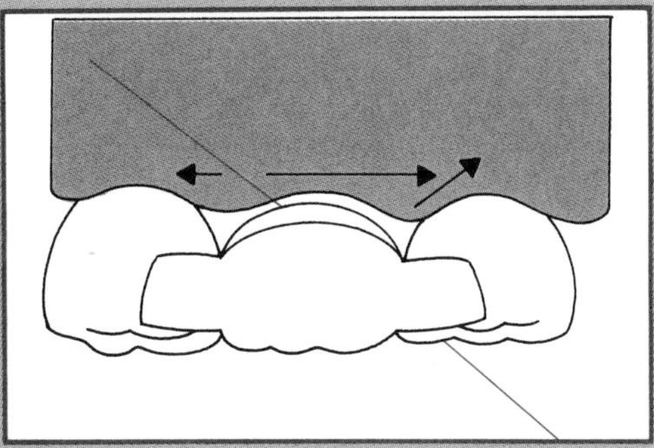

Cleaning dentures
Dentures can break or chip, so be careful not to drop them in the sink while cleaning them. An easy way to avoid danger is to partly fill the sink with water or place a towel in the bottom of the sink.

Eating with dentures
Dentures aren't as efficient for chewing as natural teeth. Your natural teeth can chew with as much as 300 lb of pressure per square inch; dentures can chew with only about 30 lb per square inch. Therefore, you may find eating difficult if you're a new denture wearer. You'll need to cut your food into smaller pieces and take smaller bites. You'll also have to learn to chew entirely on your back teeth rather than try to use your front teeth to chew, and to chew food on both sides of your mouth at the same time to equalize the pressure on your dentures.

Partial dentures

You may need a partial denture if you're missing many teeth. A partial denture is also less expensive than a fixed bridge.

A partial denture is a set of artificial teeth set in a frame, or baseplate, made of acrylic, cast metal, or alloy. (Gold frames are more flexible and easier to adjust but are also more expensive.) The size of the frame depends on the number of teeth being replaced.

The frame often has clasps that fit around healthy teeth to hold the partial denture in place. One type of partial denture connects to healthy teeth by means of an attachment device that requires no visible clasps. Many people prefer this type, although it's more expensive than other forms of partial dentures.

Partial dentures are also known as removable bridges because—unlike a fixed bridge—they can be removed. Partial dentures should be removed after each meal and cleaned thoroughly with toothpaste and a toothbrush. Brushing and flossing supporting teeth is extremely important.

While you're adjusting to new partial dentures you may want to take them out at night to give your mouth a rest. Place the dentures in a glass of water.

Even the best-fitting partial dentures loosen with repeated use and will require adjustment by your dentist or prosthodontist every few months. Proper fit is important: poorly fitted partial dentures may entrap food particles, leading to decay of the supporting teeth, and may lead to gum disease. A poor fit may even loosen the supporting teeth.

Partial denture
A partial denture can replace the missing front teeth in this mouth.

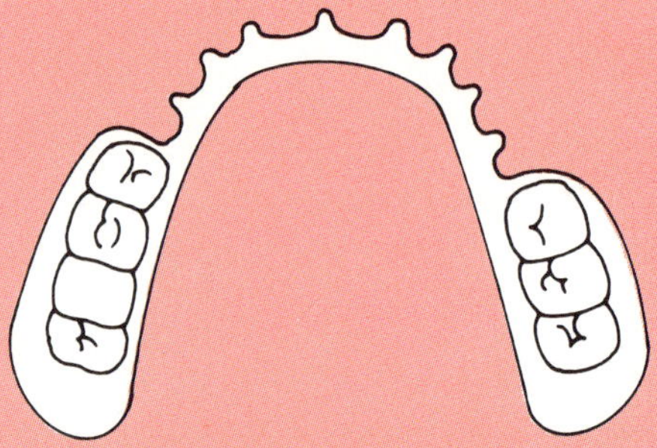

Relining dentures
Denture adhesives can provide temporary relief for loose dentures. But don't depend on adhesives for long-term use; if your dentures become loose, make an appointment with your dentist or prosthodontist to have a new base constructed. This is called relining. Your dentures will need to be relined every 3 to 4 years, and after a couple of relinings, they'll need to be completely replaced.

Some wearers of partial dentures are disturbed by the appearance of the metal clasps or hooks that connect the false teeth to the supporting teeth. The clasps can sometimes be made smaller and less visible, but not at the expense of weakening the connection between the partial dentures and the supporting teeth. Teflon "slipcovers" are now available that go over the clasps to hide them.

Full dentures

If you lose all your teeth, you'll need to be fitted with full dentures. Being fitted for dentures requires time and patience. You may need as many as eight appointments to get the correct fit. However, the end result should be natural-looking, comfortable dentures.

Losing all your teeth and being fitted for full dentures can be a traumatic experience. When your dentures are first placed in your mouth, you may notice a change in the appearance of your face. Your face may appear too small for your teeth. However, within a few weeks the facial muscles will adjust and your look will be more natural.

At first, you may experience gagging: your tongue enlarges after your teeth are removed. If you aren't fitted with dentures immediately, your enlarged tongue will be pushed back into your throat and cause gagging when you wear your new dentures. Your tongue will return to normal size after you've worn your dentures regularly for a while.

See your dentist or prosthodontist if you develop sore spots. Be sure to wear your dentures for at least 12 hours before the appointment so that the doctor will be able to detect the problem areas.

Full denture
A full denture is necessary if you lose all your natural teeth.

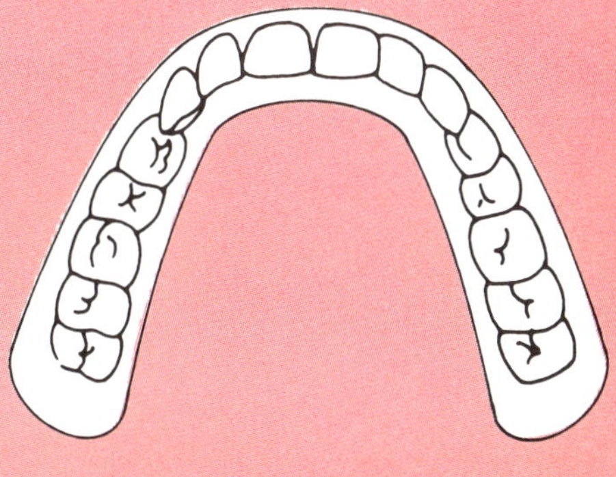

Cleaning dentures

Wear your dentures all day, every day, except when cleaning them, and clean your dentures—or at least rinse them—after each meal. Remove your dentures and massage your gums with a soft brush twice a day.

To clean your dentures, place them in a glass of water with a few drops of bleach. The bleach will reduce stains and keep your dentures smelling fresh. After soaking your dentures, brush them using a toothpaste or powder and lukewarm water. Don't use hot water—it may warp the dentures. You may want to paint disclosing solution on your dentures to see how well you're cleaning them.

Using a denture brush

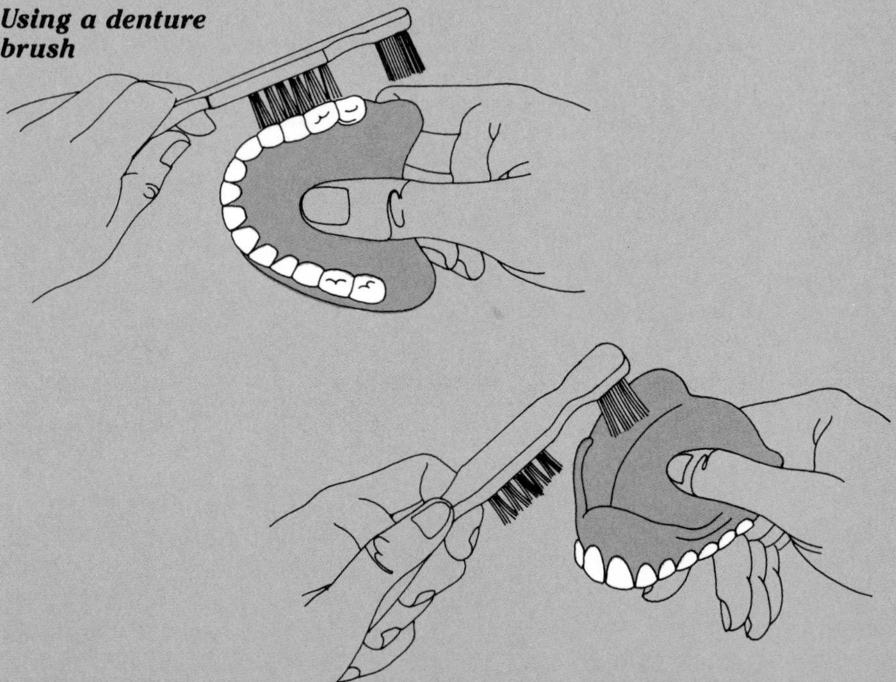

8 Coping with Pain and Emergencies

Dental phobias
Fear of pain is a major obstacle in dentistry. The American Dental Association (ADA) estimates that nearly 35 million Americans feel excessive anxiety about dentistry and that about 12 million have dental phobias—they avoid professional dental care regardless of the effects on their dental health.

Tooth problems fall into two categories: those that require immediate medical attention and those that "can wait until morning." The amount of pain is usually the determining factor.

Many dental procedures involve discomfort. Such pain is normal, and you can treat it with the measures outlined in this chapter.

If you develop sudden pain or a knocked-out tooth, you'll want to see your dentist. Tooth problems don't always occur during your dentist's normal working hours, of course. If your dentist has an answering service, you may be able to reach him at any hour. If not, you'll have to locate alternate help. If the problem is serious, contact the emergency section of your local hospital, or call a local dental clinic and ask about emergency treatment.

Pain

Most dental treatments, including a routine cleaning, can make your teeth sensitive. Afterward, you may experience pain when eating or drinking anything sweet, hot, or cold. Such pain is normal and rarely requires your dentist's special attention. The sensitivity will decrease with time. Rinsing with warm salt water may provide you temporary relief. For short-term discomfort, use aspirin or an aspirin substitute.

Pain following such dental procedures as pulling of a tooth (extraction), scraping plaque from pockets around a tooth (curettage), or root canal is also normal. Your dentist will probably give you a prescription for a pain medication to see you through the first 24 to 48 hours. However, contact your dentist if your pain and inflammation persist more than 48 hours after a root canal.

Pain and inflammation that occur soon after a dental procedure rarely involve bacterial infection; antibiotics aren't usually necessary. If the pain begins after a week or so, however, an infection is probably the cause, and antibiotics may be necessary. Take aspirin until you can visit your dentist.

How bad does it hurt?

What one person experiences as merely uncomfortable another may feel as severe pain. Before any dental procedure, ask your dentist about the pain involved. If you think you're experiencing too much pain, tell your dentist.

The extraction of wisdom teeth is usually followed by several days of pain and swelling. Rinsing with warm salt water and taking aspirin should provide some relief. However, if the pain persists and the wound doesn't heal, you may have a dry socket. A dry socket is an infection of the bone in the socket after the tooth has been removed. Such infections occur because a blood clot doesn't form and allow normal healing. See your dentist immediately; he'll scrape the socket clean to initiate fresh bleeding and allow a new blood clot to form. He'll probably prescribe antibiotics to help clear the infection.

Pain, bleeding, and swelling are normal following curettage (scraping plaque and inflamed tissue from pockets around a tooth). Take aspirin and try to eat only soft foods. If any of these symptoms seems excessive or prolonged, consult your dentist.

Pain or sensitivity in a tooth that hasn't been treated recently usually indicates the presence of decay or a lost or broken filling. Such pain can wait until morning, but see your dentist as soon as possible. Rinsing the area with warm water will keep it clean until you see your dentist.

If you experience pain from heat or from chewing, you may have a more serious condition. Sensitivity to heat may indicate that the nerve in a tooth is dying. If this condition isn't treated immediately, an infection can develop rapidly. Ice placed directly on the painful tooth may provide temporary relief.

Severe pain caused by chewing may result from deep tooth decay or a dying nerve. See your dentist immediately.

Any sudden, severe pain—whether intermittent or constant—may indicate a serious problem. You probably don't have to be told to see your dentist in such cases.

Reimplanting
To reimplant a tooth, the dentist will put the tooth back in its socket and secure it by attaching it to adjacent teeth with a wire band or by bonding. After a few weeks, the fibers on the tooth's surface should reattach themselves to the socket.

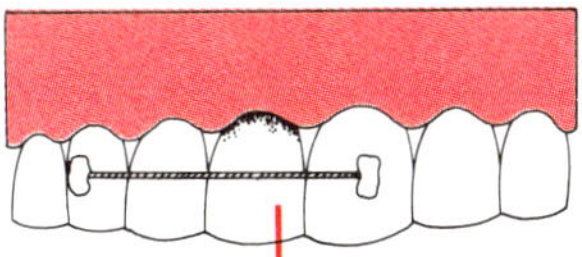

Swelling of gums
Gum swelling can be divided into two categories: swelling from an injury or dental treatment and swelling from an infection.

Swelling from an injury or dental treatment can be relieved with ice. An ice pack applied for 20 minutes on and 10 minutes off will constrict the blood vessels in the injured area and reduce the tissue fluid causing the swelling.

Swelling from an infection can be treated with heat. A heating pad, hot water bottle, or hot towel applied to your face will dilate the blood vessels and allow more blood to circulate in the infected area. Increased blood circulation brings more infection-fighting elements to the area.

Lost or broken teeth
A knocked out tooth can be put back in place—reimplanted—but immediate medical care is essential. If a tooth is knocked out, don't try to put it back in the socket. Wrap the tooth in a wet piece of gauze and hold it under your tongue (be careful not to swallow it) or put it in a small container of milk. Don't try to wash the tooth. To stop the bleeding from the socket, place a small piece of sterilized—or at least clean—gauze or tissue over the socket and bite down gently to hold it in place. The pressure will stop the bleeding. Be careful not to disturb the neighboring teeth, which may have been knocked loose or fractured by the accident.

Go to your dentist or a hospital emergency room *immediately*. A tooth can be successfully reimplanted up to about 2 hours after being knocked out. This is true for children and adults.

Fillings
Fillings that fall out or are knocked out must be replaced by your dentist. Loss of a filling can leave the tooth's nerve exposed, causing pain. Also, food may become trapped in the hole if you eat, increasing your risk of infection.

Until you get to the dentist, rinse the tooth with lukewarm water. You can relieve some of the discomfort by placing a small piece of cotton or gauze dipped in oil of cloves on the tooth.

Bridges and dentures

Don't try to repair cracked or broken bridges or dentures. You may harm both the appliance and your gums. Consider this an emergency and contact your dentist immediately.

Crowns

You're most likely to experience difficulties with temporary crowns—these may break or pop off. Call your dentist.

Permanent crowns can break or crack under stress and even under normal conditions of use. Have your dentist replace damaged crowns as soon as possible. If a crown breaks at a particularly awkward moment—such as while you're on your way to an important meeting—you may be able to hold the crown in place temporarily with petroleum jelly or denture cream.

9 Improving Your Appearance

What cosmetic dentistry can do

People have used cosmetic dentistry to:

- *make teeth squarer or rounder, wider or narrower*
- *lengthen teeth or shorten them*
- *make teeth whiter*
- *repair imperfect teeth*
- *change gum appearance.*

Your mouth is the most prominent feature of your face, and an attractive smile can go a long way toward improving your appearance. Most dental procedures are performed for reasons of dental health. However, some procedures are performed for cosmetic reasons—to improve your appearance.

Acid-etched bonding and veneering

Acid-etched bonding—usually called composite resin bonding or simply bonding—is used to repair chipped or cracked teeth, fill in gaps between teeth, cover defects in tooth enamel, and correct stained teeth. This relatively new technique usually requires no anesthetic and—unless the tooth being treated is decayed—no drilling.

Bonding can be a substitute for crowns, or caps. The procedure is less expensive than crowns and takes less time—several teeth can be bonded during one visit. Bonding is especially useful for children who fall and chip their teeth.

Your dentist will begin the procedure by separating the tooth to be bonded from your other teeth with a strip of rubber or polyester. After thoroughly cleaning and drying the tooth, he etches the tooth by applying a mild phosphoric acid solution to its surface. This acid creates microscopic pores in the tooth's surface that help composite resin bonding material adhere. The dentist then applies the composite resin—a thin, opaque plastic fluid. In the direct-bonding technique, he applies successive layers of the resin until the tooth is the desired shape and color. He then hardens the resin with a special high-intensity light (a process known as polymerization) or, if the resin is self-curing, allows it to harden naturally. When the composite resin has hardened, the dentist shapes and polishes the bonded tooth.

Bonding

In bonding, the tooth enamel is etched with a mild acid to improve adherence of the composite resin bonding material.

Layers of composite resin are brushed on and built up to the desired thickness.

Then the resin is allowed to harden naturally or is cured with a special high-intensity light, depending on the type of resin used. Bonding is often an excellent way to restore broken teeth.

Bonding is an alternative to crowns, but you may need to have the bonding repaired after 5 years. The materials used are porous and can be discolored by coffee, tea, or smoking.

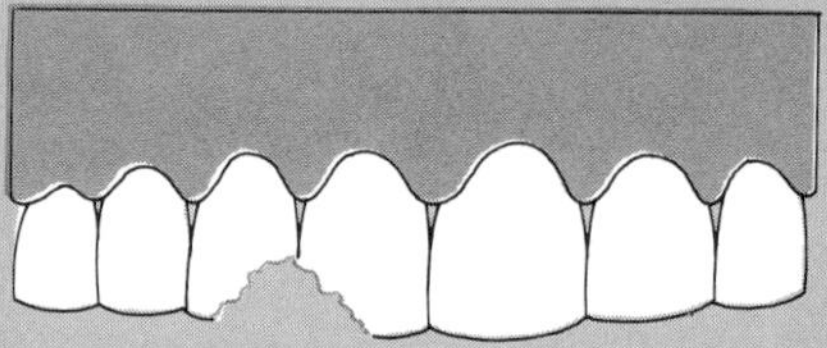

Teeth to be bonded

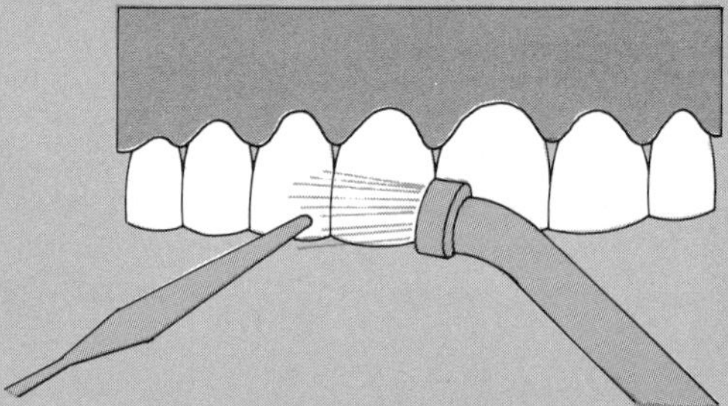

Curing the resin with high-intensity light

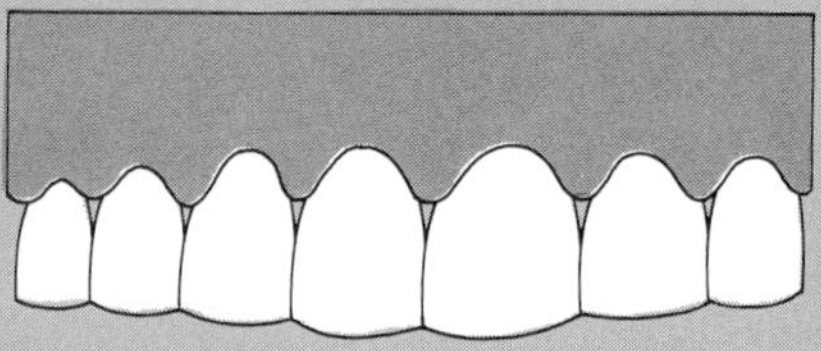

The repaired teeth

Veneering

As an alternative to the layer-by-layer buildup of direct bonding, your dentist may try veneering. In this procedure, the dentist prepares a clear veneer for the teeth. Then he coats each tooth with a resin to cover the stains. He adds a bonding material and then the prepared veneer.

If you've had veneering done, you must be careful when brushing and flossing so you don't dislodge the veneers. Also, bonding or veneering isn't recommended for repairing teeth in the back of your mouth, where chewing produces greater pressure.

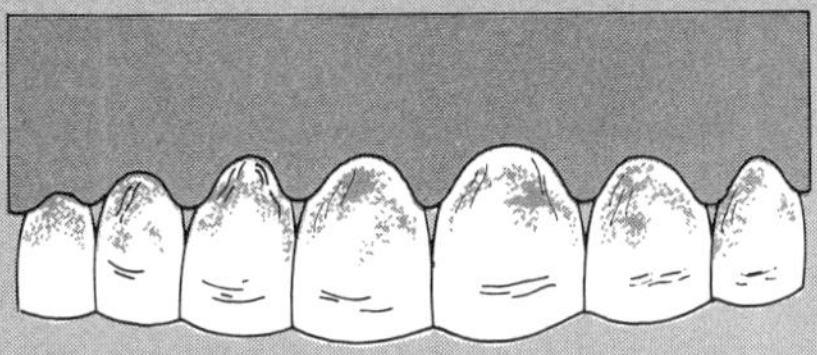

Stained teeth requiring finish

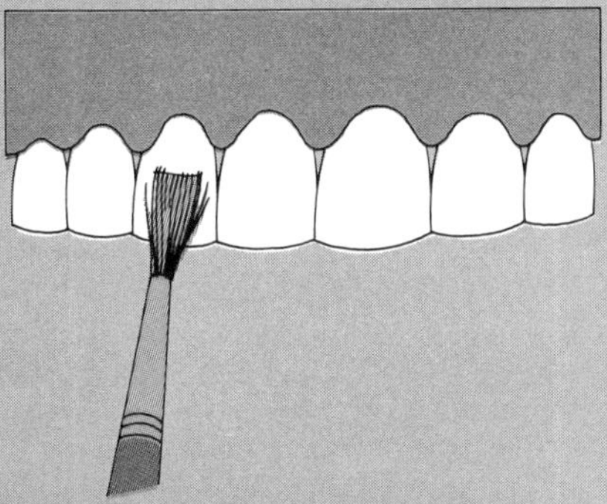

Applying resin to cover stains

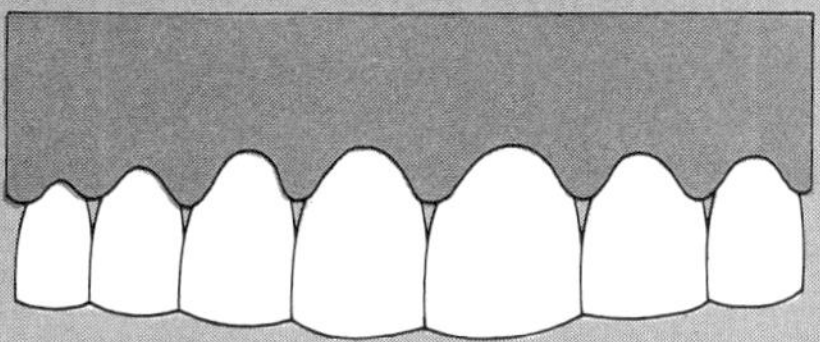

Repaired teeth with veneer in place

Children's teeth
Young teeth have a very large nerve and relatively little dentin or enamel protection, so many dentists prefer to wait until a child is at least 10 before bleaching discolored teeth.

Bleaching

Bleaching is used to lighten teeth that have become darkened. The most frequent causes of darkened teeth are from an accident—such as a blow to the jaw that results in tooth nerve damage—or use of the antibiotic tetracycline during childhood. Some teeth are naturally darker than others—this can be inherited. A child's teeth may be discolored when they erupt because of a deficiency in the enamel or an excess of fluoride in drinking water. Teeth may also become stained from tea, coffee, or tobacco. An amalgam filling in one tooth can cause discoloration in neighboring teeth.

Bleaching can lighten the color of almost all darkened or stained teeth, and the procedure doesn't damage teeth. The most common bleach is a 30% solution of hydrogen peroxide used with a controlled heat source to activate it. Each tooth is bleached separately. A tooth from which the nerve has been removed can be bleached easily, and the procedure can make quite a difference in the tooth's appearance.

Teeth that have been darkened by the use of tetracycline are more difficult to bleach. This drug reacts with calcium and can cause permanent mottling of children's teeth. Babies who haven't yet developed teeth shouldn't be given the drug; pregnant women should avoid it because unborn children can absorb the antibiotic and develop discolored teeth later in life.

Bleached-away stains may reappear within 3 months to a year after the first treatment. The teeth can be rebleached, as necessary.

Cosmetic contouring
Painless, quick, and inexpensive, cosmetic contouring can dramatically change the way you smile—and maybe the way others smile at you.

In this procedure, the teeth are marked, reshaped with dental drills or files, then finished and polished with a sandpaper disk.

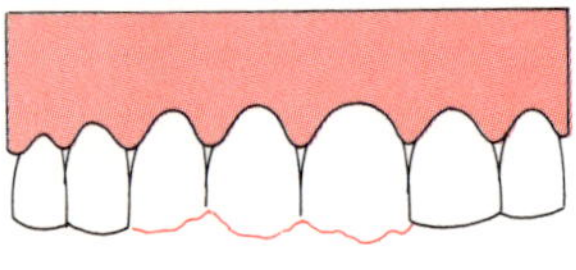

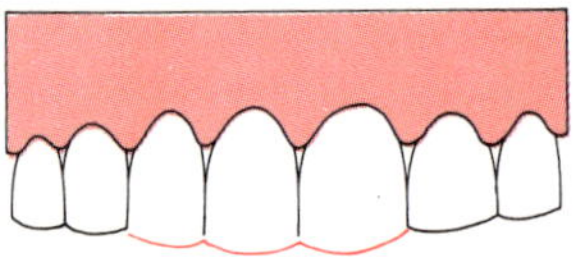

Contouring

Contouring is the reshaping of teeth to improve their appearance. This may involve making the teeth shorter, more even, or less pointed. Inexpensive contouring can produce dramatic results. Before contouring your teeth, your dentist will develop an overall view of your teeth, take measurements, use a lot of his professional judgment—and then begin to design the new shape of your smile.

What's ahead?

Prevention techniques will remain one of dentistry's main efforts, and the basic techniques shown you in this book for daily teeth and gums maintenance will probably stay the same in the immediate future. But you can look forward to additional preventive aids, such as:

- anticavity vaccines
- antibacterial chewing gum
- mouthwashes to dissolve plaque.

Wide-ranging developments, however, are probable for techniques that your dentist and other mouth-care specialists may use on patients. Here are four examples of possible advancements:

- using electrical currents to promote bone growth, heal fractures, and push fluoride beneath the tooth's surface into the dentin
- attaching a small capsule filled with fluoride to a molar to continuously release fluoride protection onto the teeth
- using laser beams to restore enamel and to smooth chips, grooves, and pits in teeth
- using braces powered by magnets or batteries to straighten teeth fast.

Index